Mother & Baby

PREGNANCY MILESTONES

CONTRIBUTING EDITOR HANNAH FOX

hamlyn

CONTENTS

LOOK OUT FOR THE TIMELINES...

to guide you along your pregnancy journey.

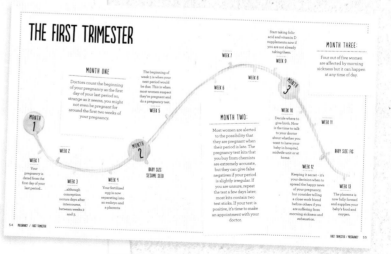

THE FIRST TRIMESTER

MONTH ONE
Doctors count the beginning of your pregnancy as the first day of your last period so, strange as it seems, you might not even be pregnant for around the first two weeks of your pregnancy.

The beginning of week 5 is when your next period would be due. This is when most women suspect they're pregnant and do a pregnancy test.

Start taking folic acid and vitamin D supplements now if you are not already taking them.

MONTH THREE:
Four out of five women are affected by morning sickness but it can happen at any time of day.

MONTH ONE
1

WEEK 1
Your pregnancy is dated from the first day of your last period.

WEEK 2

WEEK 3
...although conception occurs days after intercourse, between weeks 2 and 3.

WEEK 4
Your fertilized egg is now separating into an embryo and a placenta.

WEEK 5

WEEK 6

WEEK 7

WEEK 8

WEEK 9

MONTH TWO
2

BABY SIZE: SESAME SEED

MONTH TWO:
Most women are alerted to the possibility that they are pregnant when their period is late. The pregnancy test kits that you buy from chemists are extremely accurate, but they can give false negatives if your period is slightly irregular. If you are unsure, repeat the test a few days later; most kits contain two test sticks. If your test is positive, it's time to make an appointment with your doctor.

WEEK 10
Decide where to give birth. Now is the time to talk to your doctor about whether you want to have your baby in hospital, midwife unit or at home.

MONTH THREE
3

WEEK 11

WEEK 12
Keeping it secret – it's your decision when to spread the happy news of your pregnancy, but consider telling a close work friend before others if you are suffering from morning sickness and exhaustion.

WEEK 13
The placenta is now fully formed and supplies your baby's food and oxygen.

BABY SIZE: FIG

Mother & Baby

PREGNANCY MILESTONES

PREGNANCY

BIRTH

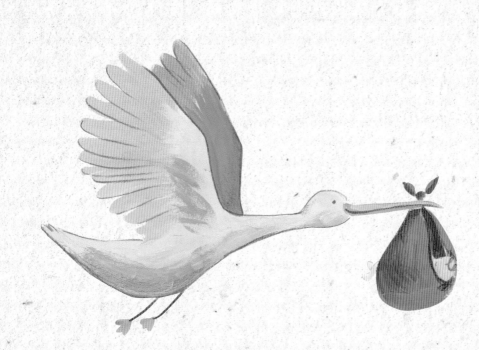

FOREWORD

Deciding to have a baby is one of the biggest decisions any woman will make and is life-changing in every way imaginable.

From the time you start trying to conceive until the precious moment you hold your little bundle of joy for the first time, you will be bombarded with a staggering amount of advice, whether it is from your mum, your best friend or the internet.

So while the journey to motherhood is an exciting experience, it is no surprise that it can also feel confusing and overwhelming as you try to work out the best choices for *you*.

At *Mother&Baby*, we have spent 60 years navigating women through pregnancy and early motherhood so our expertise is second to none. This is why we decided to put together these friendly, easy-to-read books. *Pregnancy Milestones* covers everything you need to know about pre-conception, pregnancy and birth, and for when your little bundle of joy has arrived, *Baby Milestones* is there to guide you through the exciting first year.

We are confident you will find *Pregnancy Milestones* an invaluable guide throughout your incredible journey.

Enjoy your pregnancy and beyond!

The Mother&Baby team

INTRODUCTION

You've probably picked up this book with the intention of getting pregnant or because you're recently found out you're expecting. If so congratulations! Choosing to have a baby is a monumentous decision and the start of a very exciting time!

Pregnancy Milestones lets you know what to expect from every week of your pregnancy and ensures you are armed with information about what is happening to and inside your body. We've pulled together the best experts in their fields to provide you with unparralleled, trusted and reliable guidance, information and tips on everything to do with pre-conception, pregnancy and birth. Whether it's a fertility expert to advise on the best actions to take to boost your chances of getting pregnant, a nutritionist who can provide suggestions on the ideal foods to nourish your baby, or a midwife to explain exactly why your feet have gone up a shoe size and reveal what happens when you go into labour, they're here to help and inform you.

What's more, as you'll soon discover, becoming pregnant is a bit like joining a new club that's made up of millions of other women just like you. And while we appreciate that every pregnancy is different, we also know that it helps to read about the experience of others who have been there, done that and got through it. That's why we've also included the stories of other mums to reassure you that no matter how scary, momentous or just downright weird pregnancy can be, you're not alone. There are others out there who know exactly how you feel.

The book will take you through your pregnancy on a week-by-week and month-by-month process, covering all three trimesters. But it also dedicates whole chapters to some of the really important topics so you have all the information you need at your fingertips. The book takes you from those secret first few weeks when you feel exhausted or sick and can't tell anyone, to the final days and weeks when you're making the last hurried changes to the nursery and packing your hospital bag in preparation for meeting your baby. We also cover off the many side effects of pregnancy, the tests you'll have, diet and lifestyle advice so you can nurture your baby in the best way possible, and information on what will happen during birth and in the first few days and weeks after your baby arrives.

Remember, even if this isn't your first baby, you may still find useful information, tips or answers to questions that didn't need answering first time round but are puzzling you now. We hope you find the answers right here.

Above all, we want you to be able to enjoy your pregnancy, prepare for labour and look forward to motherhood. We feel one of the best ways to do this is to be informed, as it means you can make educated choices. So whether you choose to dip into specific areas of the book, depending on where you are in your pregnancy journey, or read it from cover to cover in one night, you'll be able to find clear answers and practical tips for the many questions that will undoubtedly crop up during this time. Enjoy!

Hannah Fox,
Pregnancy specialist

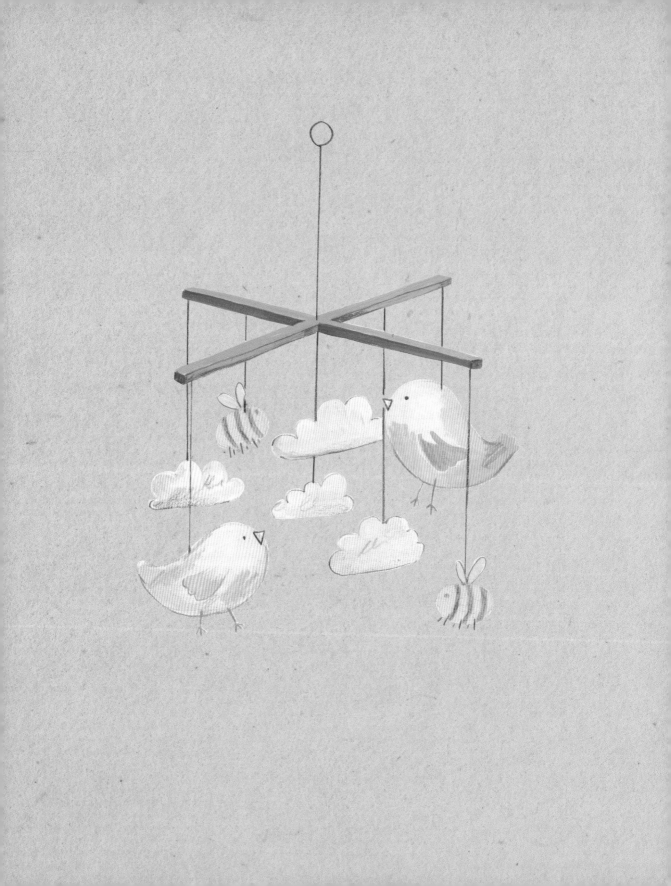

PRE-CONCEPTION

ARE YOU PHYSICALLY READY FOR A BABY?

· ·

ARE YOU EMOTIONALLY READY?

· ·

WORK OUT YOUR FINANCES

· ·

KNOW YOUR RIGHTS AT WORK AND HOW YOUR
FINANCES WILL LOOK AFTER THE BIRTH

CHAPTER ONE
ARE YOU READY FOR A BABY?

If you've picked up this book with the intention of
trying for a baby, rather than already being pregnant,
this chapter is for you. Choosing to have a baby is a
big decision – it is life-changing in every way – so it's
important that you think about certain factors in your
life before you take the plunge into parenthood.
Are you both physically and emotionally ready
for the task, and can you afford it?

AGE AND CONCEPTION — ARE YOU PHYSICALLY READY?

Despite what you've probably read in the newspapers, there's no 'right' time to have a baby, not least because you can't always choose when it will happen. You may have met the person you want to have a baby with in your teens or 20s. You might be busy developing your career and do not want a baby yet, or you may not have met the right person until later in life. So it's no surprise that the 'age issue' can leave many women worried about how it will affect their ability to conceive a baby.

Baby girls are born with a stock of around two million eggs. By puberty, this will have dropped to around 500,000 and does continue to decline. However, in spite of this massive reduction,

women are at their most fertile between the ages of 20 and 35. Fertility does begin to decline after this age simply because there are fewer eggs. Women aged 40 and over can still have babies. However, the chances of miscarriage or having a baby with chromosomal abnormalities such as Down's Syndrome, or problems such as high blood pressure during pregnancy are greater in women over the age of 35.

BECOMING A MUM — ARE YOU EMOTIONALLY READY?

The most important thing when deciding to become a parent is that you feel happy and in the right place emotionally. This might mean being in a secure and loving relationship with your partner, and/or ensuring you have plenty of friends and family around you to provide a support network.

It's vital that you and your partner are on the same page right from the start when it comes to children. Make time to talk about becoming parents long before you try to conceive. Even things that can seem miles off such as how you'll discipline your child are worth discussing at this stage so you don't get any surprises. Talk to your own mum, sister or friends who have had children. Ask them how they coped with the change.

EXPERT TIP

THE MENOPAUSE MYTH

Worried that your fertility window is closing because your mum went through menopause in her 40s? Don't. Genetics play only a part in your fertility. Other factors such as your beliefs and outlooks and your internal and external environment also play a part.

Fiona Kacz-Boulton
Fertility expert

Think about your relationship

We're led to believe all relationships should be perfect, but it's better to be realistic and look at yours as a whole. Look at every aspect of your life together: are you getting on well, do you have shared plans for the future, are you in a position to live together and bring up a child? Most importantly, avoid thinking that having a baby will cement or improve a rocky relationship. Babies can be wonderful and make you both feel closer, but the strain of looking after them can also be like a bomb going off in the relationship.

EXPERT TIP

TALK TO EACH OTHER

Communication is the base from which you'll be able to succeed as parents. Sit down with your partner and really talk about how you see yourself as parents, what you'll expect from each other and how you think you can help each other out once the baby arrives.

Dr Petra Boynton
Sex and relationships expert

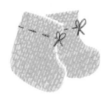

REAL LIFE

'It was my mum and sister who came through for me'

'When I discovered I was pregnant, I was living with my boyfriend and we were happy. But things deteriorated over the next few months and he moved out. I was devastated. Thankfully, my mum and sister lived nearby and stepped up to provide support for me. They came to scans and antenatal classes and helped me pick out baby items or lent me what they had. They were by my side when my daughter Maria was born and have helped me ever since. It made me realize that it doesn't matter who's in your support network, so long as there's someone to help.'

JENNY, MUM TO MARIA, FOUR

PAYING FOR A BABY – ARE YOU FINANCIALLY READY?

Babies are expensive, there's no denying it. Baby equipment can be pricey and you will be paying out for (let's face it) the next 18 years. This often accounts for the fact that many couples are deciding to having children later. That way they can work to set themselves up financially first.

You need to allow for the fact that your income will reduce while you are on maternity leave. If you are not working when you become pregnant, or have only recently started a new job, you may not qualify for maternity pay. The good news is, you can afford to have a baby, it's just a case of planning and making clever savings in the right places.

Do an audit

Work out a full budget before you think about trying for a baby. Set aside time to work out your monthly outgoings; this will show you how much money you'll have for baby items. Make a note of:

- What income you will have during your pregnancy and while on maternity leave; include any benefits you may be eligible for
- What money will come from your partner during pregnancy and for 12 months after
- Family savings that you can allocate for purchasing baby items

Start saving early on

As a rule of thumb, you should have three times the amount you need to live off each month in a savings account. That way if you can't manage on maternity leave, you can dip into your savings on a monthly basis. If you don't have enough savings, now's the time to start topping them up.

Sign up for vouchers and supermarket clubs

Get savvy with your budget once you are pregnant by joining supermarket parenting clubs as they can offer discounts on essentials such as nappies and wipes so you stock up before the birth. If you hate the idea of endless emails flooding your inbox, set up a specific 'baby deal' email address.

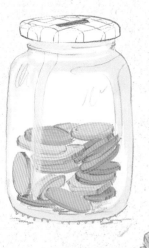

Compare prices before buying

As well as reading up on how to look after your baby, make sure you research the products you're going to buy for him or her. The more research you do – particularly with the big items such as car seats, cots and buggies – the more likely you are to pick the ones that are right for your budget and needs. Check major purchases on price-comparison sites or if you can, wait until the sales when there'll be even bigger discounts.

You may also find that friends will give you items that their children no longer need. There are local websites such as freecycle where people offer second-hand items for nothing, and you can often pick up baby bargains on sites such as eBay.

Take advantage of benefits

When you are pregnant you may also be entitled to benefits. Ask your doctor or midwife and company human resources department. Every little bit helps.

WORKING THE NUMBERS

QUESTIONS TO ASK YOUR HR DEPARTMENT

? – How many weeks before your due date do you have to tell your boss you're pregnant?

? – How many weeks of maternity leave can you take, and can you add on remaining holiday allowance on top?

? – Are you entitled to maternity pay and if so how much and for how long?

? – How many unpaid weeks of maternity leave are you entitled to? Make sure you budget for this.

CONSIDER TAKING SUPPLEMENTS
AS SOON AS POSSIBLE

....

TRY TO GET INTO GOOD EXERCISE
HABITS AS EARLY AS POSSIBLE

....

DON'T PUT TOO MUCH PRESSURE ON YOURSELF

....

THE BEST FERTILITY-BOOSTING FOODS
FOR BOTH PARTNERS

CHAPTER TWO
YOUR PRE-CONCEPTION DIET AND LIFESTYLE

Whether you're just starting out or have been struggling to conceive, it's a good idea to look at your diet and lifestyle and how it can help boost your chances of getting pregnant. The foods you eat and the way you live your life have a direct impact on the health of your body, which can, in some cases, also impact your conception chances.

A HEALTHY START

Of course, people have been getting pregnant no matter what they do, but if you're keen to take positive steps to boosting your conception chances, reassessing your lifestyle can be beneficial – plus, if you do get pregnant, you'll already be fit and well, which can only be helpful for the rest of your pregnancy.

Supplements

Once you've made the decision to start trying for a baby, you should also start taking a supplement to boost your levels of folic acid (one of the B vitamins), and eat folate-rich food (leafy green vegetables, breads and cereals). Experts say that you should be taking it before you become pregnant to reduce the risk of your baby developing spina bifida, a condition where the spinal cord doesn't form properly. Your baby's brain and spinal cord form in the first weeks of your pregnancy, when you may not even be aware that you are pregnant. It is recommended that you take 4mg folic acid daily if you are trying to conceive, and until you are 12 weeks pregnant.

Today's mass-produced food is grown in soil that's lower in nutrients than that of our grandparent's generation so it's a good idea to take a pre-conception supplement that also provides a selection of other vitamins to cover any gaps in your nutritional intake. Pick one that contains vitamins D, E, K as well as all the B vitamins. Vitamin D plays a role in biological processes in sperm and ovary cells and may affect levels of sex hormones. Supplements that contain minerals such as iodine and zinc and an amino-acid called L-Arginine may also be of benefit.

Avoid supplements containing vitamin A when you are pregnant (see page 65); you can get your dose from fruits and vegetables instead.

DID YOU KNOW?

While high amounts of caffeine aren't healthy for anyone, there are studies that claim if men have a cup of coffee before sex then their sperm is more virile.

Benefits of exercise

An active lifestyle is an important part of pre-conception health. The key is knowing your level of fitness and moderating your workouts, as excessive exercise won't do you any favours. A study in the journal *Human Reproduction* found women who performed high-frequency, high-intensity exercise had a lower rate of fertility. If you're underweight and have very low levels of fat, it can affect your periods and conception chances.

If you're already doing regular moderate exercise, this is great news as it means you can often continue (with some modifications depending on the exercise). Turn to page 76 for more tips on exercising when pregnant.

Reduce stress

Trying for a baby and not succeeding can in itself make you more stressed, so it's difficult when you're told to relax in order to improve your fertility. But the truth is that finding time to relax will definitely aid your chances. That could be by spending time with friends, taking gentle exercise to release mood-boosting endorphins, or doing a yoga or meditation class. The latter can be especially helpful as it helps to activate what is known as the parasympathetic nervous system, which is responsible for digestion and fertility.

EXPERT TIP

RELAXATION THROUGH BREATHING

The 'Sevens Breath' is a technique whereby you breathe very, very gently, quietly and slowly in for a count of seven, and then out for a count of seven. If you are struggling with this, start with five second breathing for seven cycles and build up to seven-second cycles. Focus your thoughts completely on each breath - nothing else. Stay in the present and be mindful of how the breath moves your body.

Fiona Kacz-Boulton
Fertility expert

Discuss your medication

If you plan on having a baby, but are currently taking medication, it's extremely important that you get advice from your family doctor first.

Some over-the-counter medicines and prescription drugs are safe to take while trying to conceive, others need to be adjusted. Antidepressants, for example, can also affect your libido, making you less interested in sex, which can of course further affect your chances of conceiving. If that's the case, talk to your doctor.

Other drugs that may affect conception chances include some non-steroidal anti-inflammatories (NSAIDs), steroids for conditions such as lupus, asthma or rheumatoid arthritis, thyroid medication and anti-psychotic drugs.

Q&A

'I'm currently on antidepressants but would like to have a baby. Will I need to come off them if I'm trying to conceive?'

GP **DR ELLIE CANNON** says, 'First things first, if you are on any long-term medication make an appointment with your family doctor to talk about your plans before you start trying to conceive so that he or she can work out a plan of action. If your current medication conflicts with pregnancy your doctor will look at whether the medicaton, or its dosage, can be changed, or if it's possible, try to wean you off it altogether. Your doctor will weigh up the pros and cons when it comes to taking your medication during pregnancy: do the benefits that the medication will bring you outweigh the risks of taking them during pregnancy (in which case they may be left alone), or vice versa (when changes may be possible)? Either way, the most important thing is that you don't suddenly come off your medication without talking to your doctor. He or she can help you formulate a treatment plan that works not only for pre-conception but also during pregnancy.'

Some drugs disrupt ovulation while others affect your pituitary gland, the master gland under the brain that makes some hormones and stimulates and regulates the production of others.

Look at your diet

A balanced diet that's rich in a variety of fruits, vegetables, nuts, seeds, fish and wholemeal carbohydrates, and low in processed foods will boost your health and therefore your conception chances. Given that fertility starts from within, it's worth looking at what you're putting into your body.

Watch out for processed foods, which include 'white' carbohydrates. Avoid ready meals as they can be packed with sugar, which can disrupt blood sugar and insulin levels in the body, which in turn affects hormone production. Try to eat organic meat as many commercially reared animals are given antibiotics that can interfere with hormone levels.

When it comes to alcohol, the simple truth is that your nightly glass of wine or weekend binge is not going to help your conception chances. Swedish researchers have discovered that women who drink two alcoholic beverages a day decrease their fertility chances by 60 percent. That's not to say you won't get pregnant if you do drink. The body is able to conceive if you drink alcohol. However, cutting down or cutting out booze is good for your health. Alcohol is a depressant, and will depress your energy levels just when you need as much energy as possible to help you conceive.

FERTILITY-BOOSTING FOODS

According to fertility expert Fiona Kacz-Boulton, the key to picking conception-boosting foods, is to choose ones that resemble or remind you of the male and female sex organs; as they often also contain the vital nutrients for fertility.

Male fertility boosters

Figs grow in pairs and look like testicles. Guess what Mother Nature is trying to tell us? Figs are great for sperm because of their high levels of zinc.

Bananas contain manganese, a nutrient that improves sperm quality and motility, and you don't get much more phallic than a banana.

Brazil nuts are a great source of selenium and vitamin D, which especially helps to improve male sperm.

Female fertility boosters

Avocados take nine months to form and ripen, are shaped like a womb, and rich in folic acid and monounsaturated fat, needed for regulating hormones.

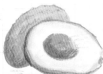

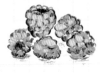

Raspberries also have a feminine shape and contain antioxidants, which help prevent damage and aging in body cells.

Coconut oil helps with healthy thyroid function and so hormonal balance.

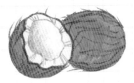

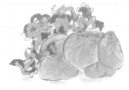

Dark green leafy vegetables such as spinach and kale are loaded with folic acid, which is needed to reduce the risk of spinal defects.

Pumpkin seeds are a source of iodine and help the cilia (the tiny hairs on cells that help the egg move down the Fallopian tube) function optimally and aid sperm mobility.

UNDERSTAND YOUR CYCLE

····································

KEEP AN EYE OUT FOR YOUR BODY'S
NATURAL SIGNS THAT YOU ARE OVULATING

····································

KNOW WHAT FERTILITY TESTS AND
CALCULATORS ARE AVAILABLE

CHAPTER THREE
UNDERSTANDING CONCEPTION

While you'll be in no doubt of the basics of how to make a baby, having an understanding of how your body works to achieve this can help when you're trying to conceive. Getting to know your menstrual cycle, for example, can help you pick the ideal time in which to have sex. While we don't want to take all the romance out of baby-making, this is useful if you're actively trying or have had trouble conceiving.

THE MENSTRUAL CYCLE

Cast your mind back to school biology lessons and you'll probably remember something about eggs, follicles, hormones and periods, but understanding how your monthly menstrual cycle prepares you to have a baby could help you become pregnant.

The process starts with the first day of your period, which is considered day one in your cycle. On day one the lining of your womb, known as the endometrium, is shed in a period. For some women, this can last a couple of days, for others, it lasts a week. And, it is your period, or the lack of it, which is often the first sign that you're pregnant.

QUICK FIX

KEEP A PERIOD DIARY

Make a note of the first day of one period to the first day on the next one; this is the length of your cycle and from this you can work out your fertility window.

Around two weeks after the first day of your period (day 14), an egg will be released by your ovary (ovulation). This egg will start to travel down one of the Fallopian tubes; this is when you are most fertile so it is the ideal time to have sex. Fertilization takes place in the Fallopian tube, so that the fertilized egg has time to start developing as it travels down the tube before it implants into the wall of your uterus.

If fertilization doesn't occur, or is too late for the egg to successfully implant into the uterus wall, the levels of progesterone and oestrogen will drop. This stimulates the production of prostaglandins that reduce the blood supply to your womb lining, causing it to break away, in what will be your period, usually 28–33 days after the first day of your last period.

Q&A

'I have irregular periods. How can I know when I should be having sex?'

Fertility expert **FIONA KACZ-BOULTON** says, 'First look at why you have irregular periods so you can try to rebalance your body (physically, mentally and emotionally). You may have irregular periods because of excessive weight gain, weight loss or stress, so you need to look at these issues. However, irregular periods can also be caused by medical conditions such as polycystic ovary syndrome (PCOS), problems with your womb or ovaries or even thyroid disorders. If there is a medical reason, you may need to see a specialist for advice on whether there's anything that can be done to help. In the meantime, I'd recommend fun, passionate sex every three days (sperm stays alive for up to five days) throughout your cycle so when you do ovulate you know your eggs will be exposed to sperm.'

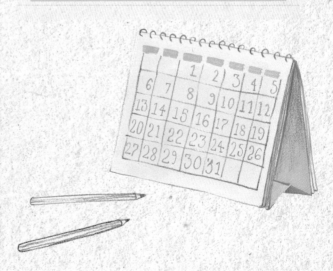

Hormone interactions

Your period begins because hormones stimulate the lining of the womb to be shed. However, a number of other hormones are triggered at the same time. The pituitary gland (see page 16) releases and regulates the levels of luteinising hormone (LH) and follicle stimulating hormone (FSH). LH and FSH stimulate your ovaries to grow one or more follicles that ripen and then release the egg within them. As a follicle develops, it triggers the production of oestrogen, which instructs the uterus to grow another womb lining. The follicle also triggers the production of progesterone, another hormone that helps to thicken the womb lining again both now and during pregnancy.

What part does the man play in this?

While all these complicated changes in your hormones are happening to allow for conception, you're probably wondering what's going on with your partner each time he's having sex. The good news for men is that, unlike women who have a finite amount of eggs that decrease every year, they continue to produce sperm for most of their life. It's what enables men to continue to become fathers well into their 60s and 70s.

Each time you have sex, your partner's sperm will stay alive inside you for a few days. If it meets an egg and successfully fertilizes that egg, you could become pregnant.

SEX FOR CONCEPTION

You may have spent most of your sex life trying to avoid having a baby, but now that you've ditched the condoms and come off the Pill or had a coil removed, it's time to start thinking about the basics of making a baby – sex – and more specifically, the best ways to boost your chances of conception.

But at the same time, it's important that sex doesn't become a chore while you're trying to conceive. Try to stay relaxed around the whole topic as much as possible, because if you become overly stressed, it could affect your fertility.

How and when?

Everybody has their own individual sex drives, and we wouldn't recommend exhausting yourself in your attempts to become pregnant; it will definitely take the fun out of sex and can increase stress. However, you can try having sex at least once a day during your most fertile period – that is the six days that stretch over the ovulation period. If you find this difficult or you don't want to spend time working out when your fertile days are, or just want to keep things simple, many experts now recommend that you simply have sex every few days throughout the month (see page 19). Remember, sperm can live for up to five days in your uterus.

While scheduling in sessions ensures that you're having sex regularly, avoid making it too mechanical. Try giving each other massages before sex so that you're feeling relaxed, change positions or move to different rooms.

KNOWING YOUR FERTILITY SIGNS

You can look out for particular signs that you're fertile each month, the main one being the changes to your cervical mucus. While we realize it's probably not something you've ever focused on before, it can be one of the easiest ways to spot when you're approaching your most fertile time.

Changing discharge

Throughout the month, the consistency of your cervical discharge changes, and it's this that reflects when you're ovulating. A clear, slippery discharge is a sign that you're fertile, mainly because it is easier for the sperm to swim through the discharge and up into the uterus. Once your discharge changes to a thicker, creamy consistency, it's harder for the sperm, which means you're less likely to conceive.

Yes, it's not something you want to be sharing over the dinner table, but a study from the University of North Carolina, USA, found that women who monitor their discharge while trying to conceive were 2.3 times more likely to conceive over a six month period than those who don't.

Mid-cycle abdominal pain

Some women say they feel a pain or cramping on either side of their lower abdomen (the site of each ovary). Known as *mittelschmerz* – a German word that means 'middle pain' – this could be a sign that you're ovulating. The pain can range from a slight twinge, to a severe cramping that lasts a few hours. You will only feel it on one side as it depends on which ovary is releasing an egg. Remember though that not every woman feels it. Also if the pain continues for longer than three days, is accompanied by vomiting and fever or you are bleeding as well, you should see a doctor immediately as this is potentially serious.

OVULATION TESTS AND CALCULATORS

These can be useful for helping you determine the best time to have sex (although don't rely on them too much or it will take all the fun out of it).

Ovulation tests work in a similar way to pregnancy tests in that they test your LH levels. LH surges just before you ovulate, indicating that it could be a good time to have sex. Most ovulation kits work by testing hormone levels in your urine and, rather like a pregnancy test, you pee on a small stick, which changes colour according to the LH level. These tests can be useful if you have an irregular cycle and so find it difficult to calculate the number of days since your last period. They are also good if your partner is away quite a bit so you can't have regular sex and you only have a few days a month when he's away for pinpointing the days when he needs to be around.

NOTES

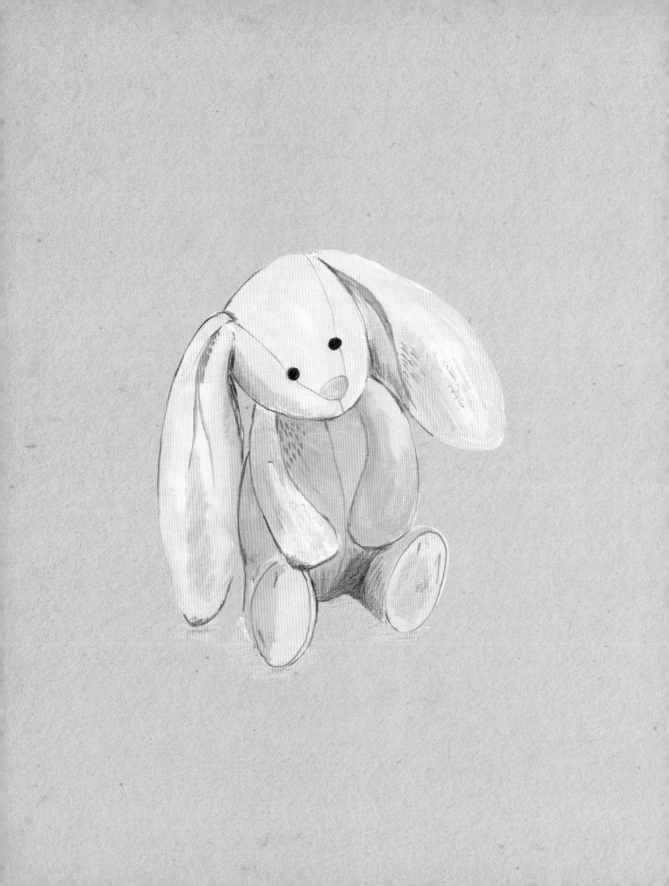

PREGNANCY

CHAPTER FOUR
FIRST TRIMESTER

This section of the book covers the first 12 weeks of your pregnancy. This stage can be a blur of secrets, interesting pregnancy symptoms, exhaustion and excitement about what's to come. But also you may not even know you're pregnant until you're at least half way through it . The prospect of actually having a baby and becoming a mother can seem strange and unreal, but luckily, you've got nine months to get used to the idea.

MONTH ONE

The first month of your pregnancy includes around two weeks when you're not even pregnant. This may sound strange, but it's because medical professionals date your pregnancy from the first day of the last period before you got pregnant.

When the lining of your uterus (known as the endometrium) is shed, your hormones start changing to allow for the release of the next egg and your uterus starts developing a new endometrium – a mixture of blood and tissue lining for a fertilized egg to implant into. Once the egg is released, usually around two weeks after the first day of your period; if the egg is fertilized (now known as a zygote) the egg cells will start multiplying as it travels along the Fallopian tube; it will implant into your womb around a week later. For the first eight weeks of pregnancy, the baby is referred to as an embryo, and after that point, it's known as a foetus.

A clever combination of hormones is now preparing your body for the pregnancy. There is one particular hormone that is very important during this process. It's known as the pregnancy hormone – human chorionic gonadotropin (or hCG), made by the cells that become the placenta – and it's the one that is picked up by pregnancy

DID YOU KNOW?

There is a window of just 24 hours for an egg to be fertilized before it breaks down. Sperm, however, can survive for a up to five days in the Fallopian tube.

Q&A

'I took a pregnancy test and it came up with a very faint line. Am I actually pregnant?'

GP **DR ELLIE CANNON** says, 'Unfortunately, you need to do another test. Pregnancy tests are designed to detect the pregnancy hormone hCG (see left) in your urine using a special stick. If only a faint line appears you may have done the test too early in your cycle or with a small quantity of urine. If this happens, wait three or four days and then repeat the test first thing in the morning when your pregnancy hormones are at their highest concentration. As with any screening test, you can of course get false positives and false negatives, so it's always a good idea to do two tests (and is why many test kits come with two sticks).

Once you have a positive result, make an appointment with your doctor so he or she can start setting up your antenatal care. During this appointment, your doctor will go through any general health problems, work out how pregnant you are (based on the first day of your last period) and therefore when your due date is, discuss your antenatal care and birthing options, and give you dietary and lifestyle advice. Some doctors repeat the pregnancy test, but this is rare as the kits they use are the same as those you can buy.'

tests. HCG starts to be released around week four so if you have a very punctual 28-day cycle and your period is late, you could take a test now and it may come up positive.

All of this will be happening with you having little or no knowledge at all. Some women claim they experience cramping around the time that the cells are implanting into the wall of the uterus. You may not get many or any symptoms in your first month, but you'll soon start to notice changes in yourself as the weeks go by.

to make sure, you can, but today's pregnancy tests are extremely accurate, so taking one or two (many tests are sold with two sticks) should let you know either way.

There are instances where you can get a false negative, usually if your period is slightly irregular and fluctuates by a few days, which can alter the hCG levels. If you get a negative result, but your period still hasn't arrived a few days later, take another test.

MONTH TWO

This is the month you are likely to discover that you are pregnant. You may be consciously having sex in order to get pregnant and using ovulation tests and so you may be ready with a pregnancy test as soon as your period is a day late. Alternatively, you may just be waiting to see what happens. Either way, once you've noticed your period is late, it's time to take a pregnancy test. This can be at different times for different women – cycles can be anything from 28 to 33 days long.

Discovering you're pregnant
Pregnancy test kits can be bought from most high street chemists and simply involve you peeing on a tab-like stick, slotting the stick back into a holder and waiting to see whether a line appears on the window, indicating that you are pregnant. Make sure you read all the instructions thoroughly before using the test – including how long you should wait before checking the result. Some tests are very technical and have a digital display that tells you how many weeks pregnant you are. However, both are essentially testing for the same thing – your levels of the pregnancy hormone hCG. If you wish to take multiple tests

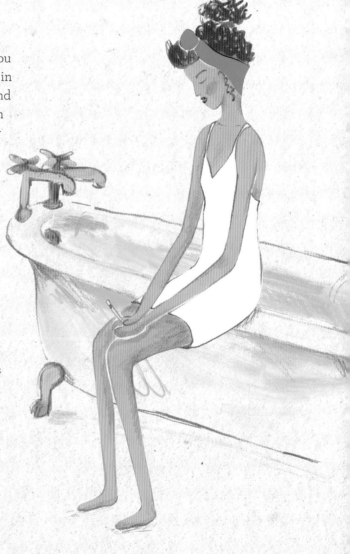

First signs of pregnancy

At this time you may start to notice other symptoms, which are quite typical of the very early days of pregnancy.

Your breasts may start to feel tender and swollen because of the surge in hormones triggered after fertilization. You may also find that you're having to pee more frequently. While normally this can be a sign of diabetes or a urinary tract infection, in pregnancy it's caused by the increase in blood flow to your kidneys, which makes them produce up to 25 per cent more urine. This increased urine production peaks towards the end of the first trimester. You will notice you need to pee more again in the final trimester, but this is more likely due to your baby squashing your bladder.

Even though you are heading to the bathroom rather frequently, don't be tempted to restrict your fluids as you need to stay hydrated for yourself and your growing baby. Avoid or reduce the number of diuretic drinks such as tea or coffee (which you'll probably be cutting down on anyway) and caffeinated soft drinks.

Taking vitamins

Ideally, you'll have begun taking folic acid and vitamin D supplements before you even started trying for a baby (see page 15), but if you haven't, then start now. Folic acid supplements (4mg daily) can still make a difference when it comes to helping to prevent your baby developing problems such as spina bifida. Vitamin D regulates calcium and phosphate in the body, both of which are needed to keep bones and teeth healthy. You should take it throughout your pregnancy (1mg daily) to provide your baby with a store for the first few months of its life. If you take a supplement, avoid one that contains vitamin A; for example anything with cod liver oil in it.

Q&A

'My breasts are so tender – what can I do?'

Midwife **HELEN TAYLOR** says, 'It's very normal to have tender breasts in the first few months of pregnancy – it is caused by the changing hormone levels in your body. You'll find that your breasts could go up by as much as two cup sizes over the course of your pregnancy. During the day, switch to soft, non-wired bras so that they don't dig into your skin. If your breasts are uncomfortable at night, try wearing soft crop tops or vest tops with added elastic support around the bust area. If you sleep on your front at this stage, try getting extra cushions to help support your breasts.'

DID YOU KNOW?

A stuffed up nose, or rhinitis of pregnancy, is common when you're expecting. Oestrogen creates an excess of mucus production, which is worsened because hormones also cause the vessels in your nose to swell, so there's less space for air and mucus to flow through.

MONTH THREE

In this month, you're nearing the time when you may want to start telling wider friends, family and your work. But for many women, this can be one of the toughest months as you get to grips with morning sickness, extreme tiredness and a gradually changing body.

Morning sickness

Not everyone gets nausea, or morning sickness, during pregnancy; it is thought to affect four out of five pregnant women. Symptoms can range from mild nausea to extreme vomiting, which can leave you weakened and exhausted.

The name morning sickness is misleading as it can affect you at any time of day. Like all the other symptoms it's caused by the extra pregnancy hormones circulating in your body. The good news is that for many women (although not all), morning sickness eases as they enter the second trimester. Until then, there are different things you can do to alleviate the problem.

Snack on plain foods

Sometimes the only thing that can make you feel better when you're feeling sick is food. Keep the foods plain, oatcakes or crackers are good, so they don't over-stimulate your stomach. It's a good idea to keep a snack by your bedside table so you can eat before you get up as that can sometimes alleviate early morning nausea.

Try ginger and mint

Both ginger and mint are natural stomach settlers, so consider eating a ginger biscuit or drinking a peppermint tea if you're feeling unwell.

Acupressure

Some women are helped by acupressure – a therapy where specific pressure points around the body are pressed or massaged to alleviate health problems. Make sure you go to a qualified therapist who treats pregnant women. Alternatively, try acupressure wrist bands, which apply pressure to an area of the wrist to help ease the nausea.

Sipping drinks or sucking ice lollies can help

It's important to keep your fluid levels up if you're throwing up regularly. But if drinking from a cup is stimulating your gag reflex, try sucking on an ice lolly. They're not only refreshing but also hydrating. You can also try sipping fluids through a straw so you don't have to swallow too much liquid in one go.

Coping with the tiredness

There's feeling sleepy from one too many late nights watching films or seeing friends, and then there's the all-encompassing exhaustion that often characterizes early pregnancy. This can be a very difficult time especially if you're trying to keep your pregnancy a secret, but struggling to carry on as normal.

Don't put pressure on yourself to continue with your usual social activities; your body is working hard to adapt to pregnancy. If you're struggling, try getting outside for at least 20 minutes a day. A brisk walk in the fresh air can actually help to boost energy levels as it raises circulation

DID YOU KNOW?

Extreme pregnancy sickness – known as hyperemesis gravidarum – affects about 3% of women and can be extremely debilitating. If you're struggling to keep any food or fluids down, see your doctor who may be able to prescribe special anti-sickness medication.

and increases the amount of oxygen reaching your brain. You could also try using an invigorating shower scrub each morning to wake you up – try one with citrus fruits and finish with a blast of cool water. Have a nap when you get home from work to boost your energy for the evening. The good news is that the tiredness often eases as you go into the second trimester.

WHEN TO ANNOUNCE YOUR PREGNANCY

If you're struggling with morning sickness, falling asleep in the work toilets and concerned that people might notice your bump developing, it's understandable that you may worry people will guess that you are pregnant before you're ready to tell them. It can help to have one 'buddy' at work who you can share your secret with. He or she can help cover for you if you're having a tough morning or don't want to be seen avoiding alcohol at an office social event.

As for telling parents and relatives, it can be a bit of a minefield if you speak to one set of in-laws before the other. It might be worth trying to bring them all together for a lunch so you can announce it to both at the same time. Whenever you do, brace yourself for *lots* of unsolicited advice.

Beware of social media announcements as not everyone is on Facebook so putting a picture of your scan up may only get the message to some of your friends and family, especially if your great aunt Iris isn't on social media.

When it comes to your employers, find out when you are obliged to tell them; it may not be until quite late but this depends on your job as they may need to alter your working pattern. Bear in mind that your boss might not be as overjoyed as you are, as arranging cover for maternity leave can be a challenge. However, they are not allowed to discriminate because you're expecting.

REAL LIFE

'I told my family on my birthday dinner'

'After trying for a baby for nearly a year, I was thrilled when I finally became pregnant. I was desperate to tell people, but my husband and I decided to wait until we'd had our first scan. This was easy with our family – my birthday was a week after the scan, so we gathered everyone together and told them over the dinner. Work was a little trickier as I had terrible nausea and looked permanently tired. The girl I sat next to is a great friend and I think she twigged because she kept asking if I was ok. I ended up telling her and swearing her to secrecy, but it worked out well as she covered for me and bought me non-alcoholic drinks if we were out.'

LUISA, MUM TO OLIVER, 16 MONTHS

APPOINTMENTS, SCANS AND TESTS

Now that you've told your family doctor that you're pregnant, he or she will have referred you to your chosen hospital and antenatal care team. You'll have your first official booking in appointment with your midwife at around 10 weeks. She will talk to you about your options (see opposite) and arrange your first scan. In some areas, you may have an early scan at around six to eight weeks to confirm pregnancy, particularly if you've experienced bleeding, and to check everything is developing well. This is usually done using a transvaginal probe.

Your 12-week scan

Although it's often called a 12-week scan, this can be done any time between 11 and 13 weeks. This scan is a landmark moment as it's the first time parents see their baby (or babies), and it makes everything feel a lot more real.

How do scans work?

An ultrasound machine emits high-frequency soundwaves through a hand-held device called a transducer. The soundwaves bounce off solid objects such as bone and tissue, but pass through fluids, and the 'echoes' are converted into an image on a screen. The sonographer will put special conductive gel over your stomach and then run the transducer over it to get an image. The quality of ultrasound machines these days means that you *don't* have to drink pints of water beforehand. However, if he or she is struggling to see something, you may be asked to drink something during the session as fluid in your bladder helps give a clearer view of the uterus.

The sonographer will measure your baby, check the anatomy as far as possible at this early stage (checking the skull, brain, arms, legs, the heart, stomach, bowel, pelvis and bladder). Once all the

measurements and checks have been done, you can usually request a print out of the scan to take home. Most hospitals will charge you for this.

Depending on your age and initial blood tests (see opposite) you may be offered a nuchal translucency scan first, to check for risk of chromosomal abnormalities such as Down's syndrome. This scan measures the thickness of the pocket of fluid at the back of your baby's neck. The more fluid there is, the higher the risk.

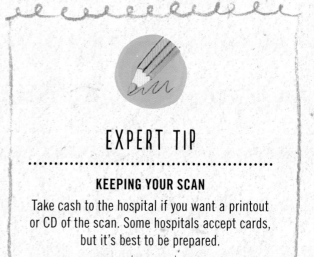

EXPERT TIP

KEEPING YOUR SCAN

Take cash to the hospital if you want a printout or CD of the scan. Some hospitals accept cards, but it's best to be prepared.

Helen Taylor
Midwife

YOUR BOOKING IN APPOINTMENT

During this appointment, you'll meet with
your midwife and he or she will:

- Give you your maternity notes and care plan – you'll need to bring these notes to each appointment.

- Identify any potential risks associated with any work you may do such as heavy lifting or working with chemicals.

- Measure your height and weight and calculate your body mass index (BMI). This is to see if you're overweight and so at an increased risk of gestational (pregnancy) diabetes.

- Measure your blood pressure and test your urine for protein. The latter can be a sign that you have an infection or a condition called pre-eclampsia, which can be dangerous for you and your baby. These will be repeated at every check-up.

- Offer you screening tests and make sure you understand what is involved before you decide to have any of them. These screening tests will check your blood group and rhesus status (see page 83 for more on this), check if you have hepatitis B and C, a susceptibility for rubella (German measles – which can be very serious in pregnancy), syphilis and HIV. An initial blood test can also check if you carry a risk of having a baby with Down's Syndrome (which can then be confirmed through further checks).

- Offer and book you in for ultrasound scan at 11 to 13 weeks to calculate your baby's due date and another one at 18 to 22 weeks (your 20-week anomaly scan) to check the development of your baby and screen for abnormalities.

ADDITIONAL SCANS AND TESTS

During your initial antenatal screening tests, you'll have had a blood test and had the nuchal fold (an area at the back of your baby's neck that holds liquid) measured during the ultrasound. This is to check for the likelihood of whether your baby will be born with chromosomal anomalies linked to Down's, Edwards' or Patau's Syndrome. Down's, Edwards' and Patau's syndromes are all conditions caused when the cells in our bodies have an extra copy of a particular chromosome. For Down's Syndrome it is chromosome 21, for Edwards' it is chromosome 18 and for Patau's it is chromosome 13. The latter two are very serious conditions and chances of survival during pregnancy or in the days after birth are very low. However, babies born with Down's Syndrome, while experiencing some mental and physical disabilities, can go on to lead very full and happy lives.

If, from your initial tests, it is discovered that your risk of having a baby born with these conditions is considered to be greater than 1 in 150 you will be offered either a chorionic villus sampling (CVS) or an amniocentesis test. To put this into context, 95 per cent of tests will show a lower risk of chromosomal abnormalities and only 5 per cent will be higher risk. However, the risk does go up as you get older.

Chorionic villus sampling (CVS)

You can be offered a CVS test from 10 weeks, but it's usually done between 11 and 14 weeks of pregnancy. During the procedure, a very fine needle is inserted into your uterus (using an ultrasound machine as a guide) to remove a small amount of tissue from your placenta. The tissue contains cells which will have the same DNA as your baby, and so can be tested for

conditions such as Down's Syndrome. The test carries a small risk of miscarriage (of about 2 per cent) and infection, which is why it will only be carried out if your initial screening tests show a higher than normal risk.

Amniocentesis

This is generally carried out later into your pregnancy – at around 15 weeks. The advantage is that the chances of miscarriage are lower (around 1 per cent). For this procedure, a needle is once again inserted into your uterus, but this time a sample of amniotic fluid is taken. It contains cells shed from the foetus that can be examined and tested for a number of conditions, including those mentioned above.

Once the samples have been analyzed, your doctor will discuss the results with you and let you know if they have come back positive or negative. Most are negative, so try not to worry too much. If they do come back positive, you will be offered counselling on what your next options are, including deciding to carry on with the pregnancy (and what that will involve) or choosing to terminate it.

Non-Invasive Prenatal Testing (NIPT) for Down's syndrome

These are relatively new tests, which analyze samples of foetal DNA found in the mother's blood. It means they don't need to use the invasive methods of CVS and amniocentesis, which carry risks. The blood test is thought to be 99 per cent accurate. However, in many cases, these tests are only available to people who pay privately, and are not always available to those receiving state-funded care.

·································

'Is there a set amount of antenatal check-ups that you get during pregnancy?'

Midwife **HELEN TAYLOR** says, 'On the basis of a normal pregnancy, state hospitals usually offer approximately ten pregnancy appointments (slightly fewer for second-time mums) and two scans (at around 12 and 20 weeks). After the initial booking in appointment, a routine midwife check-up will involve taking your blood pressure, a urine test, and abdominal palpation – measuring the growth of your bump – and checking how the baby is lying (which is most relevant when near your due date) as well as listening in to foetal heartbeat. These are usually quite short (around 12–15 minutes). If you opt for an independent midwife, appointments are generally longer to allow plenty of time to answer any questions you may have.'

Scheduled appointments

Generally, you'll have appointments with your midwife at the following times:

- Eight to 12 weeks – booking in appointment. You'll have a blood test to check for rubella, syphilis, hepatitis B, rhesus status, anaemia and Down's Syndrome risk. The midwife will check your blood pressure and test your urine for protein, and take a full health history.

- Eight to 14 weeks – dating scan (see page 32).
- 16 weeks – review, discuss and record the results of any screening tests, measure your blood pressure and test your urine for protein.
- 18-20 weeks – anomaly scan.
- 25 weeks – measure the size of your uterus, check your blood pressure and test your urine for protein. You will only have this appointment if this is your first baby.
- 28 weeks – measure the size of your uterus, check your blood pressure and test your urine for protein. You'll also be offered blood tests to check you're not anaemic or developing gestational diabetes.
- 31 weeks – measure the size of your uterus, check your blood pressure and test your urine for protein. Discuss the results of the tests you had at 28 weeks. You will only have this appointment if this is your first baby.
- 34 weeks – measure the size of your uterus, check your blood pressure and test your urine for protein.
- 36 weeks – measure the size of your uterus and check the position of your baby, check your blood pressure and test your urine for protein.
- 38 weeks – measure the size of your uterus, check your blood pressure and test your urine for protein.
- 40 weeks – measure the size of your uterus, check your blood pressure and test your urine for protein. You will also be given information about what will happen if you go overdue. You will only have this appointment if this is your first baby.
- 41 weeks – measure the size of your uterus, check your blood pressure and test your urine for protein. You will be offered a membrane sweep and he or she will discuss the options and choices about being induced.

WHICH FOODS BEST HELP YOU
MANAGE YOUR SIDE EFFECTS

MANAGE YOUR ACHES AND PAINS

PERK UP YOUR MOOD AND COMBAT TIREDNESS

KNOW THE REAL RED FLAGS DURING
PREGNANCY AND WHEN TO SEEK
PROFESSIONAL HELP

CHAPTER FIVE
SIDE EFFECTS AND
SYMPTOMS OF PREGNANCY

With your body going through such amazing
changes as it makes your baby, it should come as
no surprise that you'll start noticing many new
things – and we're not just talking about your
bump. While they can be surprising, frustrating,
or just downright weird, there's usually a way of
managing them. Here's what you may (or may not)
experience over the next nine months.

ABDOMINAL CHANGES

As your baby grows and your uterus widens, it will start putting pressure on your other organs, in particular your stomach, bowel and bladder. In addition, certain pregancy hormones prepare you for pregnancy and birth, which can cause changes too. All this can affect you in numerous ways.

What is heartburn?

So called heartburn actually has nothing to do with your heart. It is in fact a form of indigestion and one of the most common complaints during pregnancy; 80 per cent of women experience it at some point. A burning sensation after you eat is the most obvious sign. For some this can start just a few weeks into pregnancy. For others, it becomes a problem later on when their bump is expanding, restricting the space for the stomach.

One of the hormones released in pregnancy, relaxin, helps loosen the muscles and ligaments in the body to prepare for your baby's arrival. But it also relaxes the muscles at the point where your gullet, or oesophagus, enters the stomach. The burning sensation results when the acid in your stomach rises up through the muscles and causes irritation. Your expanding womb can also press upwards on your stomach, forcing the acidic contents up towards this opening.

Luckily antacids, or indigestion medication, are one of the few medicines that are safe to take during pregnancy. The liquid ones are best. Eat small and regular meals – it's better to eat six little plates of food through the day rather than three large ones. Avoid eating late at night because when you lie down it makes it easier for your stomach contents to rise up and cause discomfort. You could also try drinking a glass of milk or having some yogurt as it can have a cooling effect, although bear in mind that dairy products can make some people's symptoms worse.

Urinary tract infections (UTIs)

If you've been feeling uncomfortable each time you go for a pee, it could be a sign of a urinary tract infection (UTI), a common problem during pregnancy. A UTI is caused by bacteria in your lower urinary tract, or urethra (the short tube that runs between your bladder and the hole that you pee out of).

In pregnancy, hormones change the balance of bacteria in your body, which when combined with a slightly compromised immune system during pregnancy, make you more prone to picking up infections. Plus, pregnancy hormones relax the muscles surrounding the tubes connecting your kidneys and bladder, slowing down the flow of liquid between the two . This can allow bacteria to grow before it's flushed out.

Typical symptoms include feeling like you need to wee (but not managing to do so), a burning or stinging sensation when you do urinate and pain in the bladder area. If you think you might have a UTI, see your doctor because untreated it could

QUICK FIX

. . . .

AVOID HEARTBURN

Keep a food diary. Note down any foods that trigger heartburn to remind you to avoid them. Common culprits are fizzy or caffeinated drinks, fruit juice, tomato-based sauces, curry or rich, fatty foods.

lead to a kidney infection, which is dangerous for your baby. Your doctor will prescribe antibiotics safe for pregnancy to treat the infection and your symptoms should clear up in a couple of days.

There are over-the-counter remedies that can ease the symptoms such as sachets of powder containing sodium citrate, which reduces the acidity of your urine so it's not as painful when you pee. Drink plenty of fluids – some women swear by cranberry juice – to flush out the

infection and make sure you wipe yourself from front to back when going to the toilet as that will reduce the chances of bacteria entering your urinary tract in the first place.

Incontinence

At the other end of the scale lies incontinence. Rather than not being able to pee, you may find yourself not being able to stop yourself. It's caused by one of two things depending on the stage of your pregnancy – hormones in the first weeks (especially hCG), and later the pressure of your baby pushing on your bladder. Once again the hormone relaxin is partly to blame as it can also affect the pelvic floor muscles that control the flow of urine. As your baby grows, he'll push down on your bladder, making it harder for you to hold in large amounts of urine.

Piles

This is actually the inflammation of veins in or around the lower rectum and anus. Also known as haemorrhoids, piles can occur at any time, but they are common during pregnancy because the hormones rushing around your body cause your veins to relax. They can also be caused by straining too much when you go to the loo (often

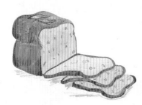

REAL LIFE

'My piles felt itchy and uncomfortable'

'When I became pregnant I found I was getting constipated quite regularly. One day I noticed blood on the tissue after doing a poo. Naturally, I was terrified that it was something to do with my baby, so I called my family doctor and got an appointment that day. She examined me and explained that I had piles, and told me that they were quite common during pregnancy. I'd never heard of piles before. She explained what they were and told me to use an over-the-counter cream to ease the itching and to make sure I ate a fibre-rich diet. They flared up throughout my pregnancy, but have disappeared since.'

PHILIPPA, MUM TO BILLY, 13 MONTHS

because you're constipated) or from the weight of your baby putting pressure on the veins. The pressure forces the vein walls to bulge out and fill with blood, causing small bumps, which can appear just inside the anus.

Going to the toilet can push piles outside the body and you may be able to feel them. They can feel itchy or the area can be quite sore – particularly when passing faeces. The veins may bleed a little – it will appear as bright, red blood on the toilet tissue or in the bowl. If you think you have piles, you're not sure where the blood is coming from, or it is very dark red or black, talk to your doctor.

While you can't instantly get rid of piles, there are lots of ways to reduce the effects, including sticking to a healthy high-fibre diet to prevent constipation. Make sure you gradually add fibre to your diet and keep your fluids up, otherwise you may become more constipated, making the situation worse. Try pressing a cloth wrung out in ice water against the piles to soothe the pain. If nothing seems to be easing your discomfort, see your doctor who may prescribe medicines and ointments to help soothe the inflammation.

Excess gas

You're probably thinking, 'great, this is the last thing I need'. Unfortunately, being rather gassy is an extremely common symptom of pregnancy. Pregnancy hormones are the culprit once again, this time it's because they slow down your digestive system. As a result there's more time for the bacteria in the waste food to produce gas, and this can become trapped in your stomach or intestines. The result is that you may find yourself needing to burp and passing wind just when you least want to or expect it. Combined with the looser muscles throughout your body because of hormones, you could find it's also much harder to hold excess gas in when you want to.

Q&A

'I've been feeling quite constipated and have started eating more roughage and bran in my diet but it's not working. What can I do?'

Nutritionist **CHARLOTTE STIRLING-REED** says, 'While eating plenty of high-fibre food such as whole wheat cereals can help to prevent constipation in pregnancy, it only works if you also drink plenty of fluids. Things like oats and bran help to make your stools bulky, so they're easy to pass, but you also need fluids so that they're soft. Drink at least 2 litres (3½ pints) of fluid a day, water and herbal teas are the best choices during pregnancy to ensure it's easier for you to go. Also, try not to increase your dietary fibre by too much too quickly. Introduce it gradually, especially if your diet is very low in fibre to begin with.'

Don't worry too much if you let one slip. Most people won't notice, and if they do you've got the perfect excuse – you're pregnant. If you're worried, go easy on fizzy drinks – even carbonated water, and avoid known gassy foods such as cabbage, sprouts or beans.

ACHES AND PAINS

When you're carrying an ever-growing bump around with you all day, you can develop aches around your body. While they can be uncomfortable, most disappear after the birth.

Pelvic pain

Normally, your pelvis is locked into a secure position, but pregnancy can trigger a condition known as pelvic girdle pain (PGP). In the past it was suggested that hormones loosened tendons around the pelvis causing instability, but the latest research suggests it's caused by a pre-existing pelvic joint problem. The pelvis has three joints and if one becomes stiff and stops moving properly, it causes irritation and muscle tightness in the others as they have to compensate.

PGP is more likely to flare up if you have a history of back pain, are overweight, have had a fall or pelvis injury, don't sit properly at your desk (read: slouch and cross your legs) or are a second- or third-time mum. If you suffered with PGP in a previous pregnancy, you may find it's worse in the next one. Typical

DID YOU KNOW?

Pelvic girdle pain was often known as symphysis pubis dysfunction (SPD), but this term has fallen out of favour as that only refers to pain at the front of the pelvis. PGP is the umbrella term for all pain in the pelvis.

symptoms include pain, and sometimes a clicking or grinding sensation in the pelvic area. You may also find it difficult walking and it can be extra painful during sex or when you place all your weight on one leg.

Talk to your midwife or doctor. Either can refer you to a physiotherpist who may be able to manipulate the joints to mobilize them. He or she will prescribe stability exercises and stretches, and give you general advice about posture. You can also wear special belts and tubigrips can also be used to support the joints. Exercise in water can help strengthen the muscles around the pelvis.

Back ache

This is one of the most common symptoms of pregnancy, especially in the later stages as your bump gets bigger. It affects up to 75 per cent of pregnant women at some point. Back ache generally occurs for two reasons – the first is the extra weight of your bump changes your centre of gravity, which can put strain on your spine. The second is the hormone relaxin, which not only helps to make ligaments in the pelvis looser so your baby can be delivered, but it can also destabilize joints throughout the rest of your body, which can put pressure on your back. Lower back they are particularly common in pregnancy. Nobody is entirely sure what causes them, but some experts believe it's a shortage of nutrients such as calcium and magnesium being available to your body because they're being used to grow your baby.

Cramps are most likely to occur when you've been sitting or lying still for a while, so don't be surprised if you're woken up at night by them. Try some yoga stretches (straightening out your leg and flexing your ankle and toes). You could also get your partner to massage the affected muscle.

Restless legs are exactly that – you feel as if you can't keep your leg still. It can be quite disconcerting, but isn't usually painful in the way leg cramps are. While it can affect both men and women, around one in four mums-to-be will develop it. Experts aren't sure what causes restless legs, but it's not harmful to your pregnancy or baby's health. There's no specific cure for the condition, so it's often a case of trial and error about what – if anything – will ease the symptoms. Some women report a warm bath, gentle massage or hot water bottle resting on the legs can help. If you've developed the condition during pregnancy, it'll probably disappear once your baby arrives.

pain is the most common. Upper back problems are less common and are usually connected to the way your baby is lying. Some woman have found visiting a chiropractor or osteopath who specializes in treating pregnant women can help. If you spend a lot of time sitting, try to give yourself regular breaks, and ensure that when you do sit, your hips are higher than or level with your knees. You could also try wearing a supportive bump band to help relieve the weight that's pulling your spine forward.

Leg cramps and restless legs

If, while lying in bed at night, you suddenly feel your calf muscle spasm, it's most likely to be leg cramps. They can happen to anyone, but

QUICK FIX

BEDTIME SNACKS

To prevent night cramps, tuck into snacks that contain calcium and magnesium, such as a glass of milk and a banana, as those nutrients are thought to reduce the likelihood of cramps.

TIREDNESS AND MOOD SWINGS

Are you struggling to get to sleep sometimes and feeling like a zombie during the day? You're not alone. Tiredness and insomnia are one of the most common side-effects of pregnancy and can occur throughout the nine months, but can be particularly acute in the first and third trimester.

Tiredness

You may start feeling tired as early as six or seven weeks into your pregnancy. It makes sense as at this stage, your body is very busy making the placenta and developing your baby. Plus, your hormone levels and metabolism are changing fast and you tend to have lower blood sugar and blood pressure levels, all of which can leave you feeling completely exhausted.

It can be hard if you're a bit of a night owl, or like to squeeze in lots of post-work activities, and now find yourself falling asleep in front of the TV every night. But take heart from the fact that the first trimester tiredness tends to ease by about 12–14 weeks and you may get a burst of energy as you enter your second trimester. In the meantime don't push yourself; put your feet up in the early evening if you need to. Your body is working overtime and needs time to recover.

However, you are likely to find yourself getting tired again as you near the end of your pregnancy, mainly because by this time you'll be carrying a sizeable bump around – and it grows bigger every day. With any luck, you'll be about to, or have just gone on maternity leave, so at least you are not working. Make the most of this time to pamper yourself, take daytime naps and relax as much possible. We know it's tempting to spend those last few weeks rushing around getting everything for your baby but it's important to take time out for yourself as well to prepare for the weeks ahead.

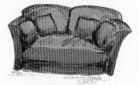

REAL LIFE

'I was asleep on the sofa by 7pm every night'

'My first trimester was a blur of extreme tiredness. Although I was lucky to get away with only mild nausea, the exhaustion took me completely by surprise. It started a week or two after I found out I was pregnant and continued until I was about 14 weeks. Getting up in the morning felt like the biggest chore, I was totally spaced out at work and would fall asleep on my train commute home. My partner was great and totally understanding about how I felt. I tried to have a decent lunch at work so I could grab a really quick snack in the evening and then head straight to bed. I was relieved when I got my energy back in my second trimester.'

EMILY, MUM TO RACHEL, FOUR MONTHS

DID YOU KNOW?

According to the National Sleep Foundation in the UK, 78 per cent of women experience disturbed sleep in pregnancy.

Watch out for anaemia

Your body needs iron to make red blood cells (haemoglobin), and at the moment your body is making more red blood cells than before. Low iron stores cause anaemia and it can be another reason you may be feeling tired. Although your daily requirement for iron (14.8mg) doesn't go up in pregnancy, anaemia tends to be more obvious at this time because your body is working harder and you're having regular blood tests. And at this stage, it's vital that you have healthy iron levels as your body is making more blood to help in the growth and development of your baby.

As well as tiredness, anaemia can cause breathlessness, palpitations and pale nail beds and eyelids so talk to your midwife at your next appointment if you're worried. You can take iron supplements (although they can cause constipation – see page 66) but it's a good idea to incease your dietary intake of iron-rich food such as red meat and poultry, pulses, dried fruit, fortified cereals and green leafy vegetables.

Dizzy spells

Have you experienced head rushes or are you generally feeling a bit wobbly since becoming pregnant? Dizzy spells can occur in pregnancy for different reasons, but often it's related to either anaemia (above) or blood pressure problems.

Your blood pressure could be either too low or too high, as either can make you feel slightly faint. While it's a common problem, you should always talk to your family doctor or midwife about it because it can be quite significant.

Remember too that if you've been feeling very unwell with nausea and sickness, that could also make you feel dizzy and/or faint, especially if you haven't been able to keep much food down. Talk to your doctor or midwife if necessary.

Not getting enough sleep

Whether it's worrying about the prospect of becoming a mum or the endless middle-of-the-night trips to the loo, it's not always easy to get a full night's sleep when you are pregnant. Factor in trouble finding a comfortable sleep position thanks to your growing bump and coping with heartburn (see page 37) and it's no wonder you're nodding off in your 9am meeting.

Create a sleep-inducing space in your bedroom by banning all electronic items and turning off phones. They emit a blue light that actually prevents the release of the sleep-inducing hormones seratonin (which calms you down and regulates sleep) and melatonin (which regulates your sleep pattern). Make sure the room isn't too hot and bank up your bed with different pillows so your head is slightly raised; this reduces the problems of heartburn, which can keep you awake. You could invest in a specially shaped pregnancy pillow, which will support your bump as you lie on your side (always your left) and support your knees to ease backache and pelvic discomfort.

If you're waking in the night with nausea (trust us, this isn't restricted to morning), keep a small snack by your bed. A banana or oat cereal bar are good as both contain tryptophan, a neurotransmitter, which triggers seratonin.

If getting up for the loo is disturbing your sleep, don't avoid fluids completely. Sip smaller amounts more regularly in the evening and allow plenty of toilet trips before you head to bed.

Q&A

'I'm in my third trimester and every time I wake up it takes ages to go back to sleep. Any advice?'

Doula **MIA SCOTLAND** says, 'In the third trimester, it's common to find it more difficult to sleep through. Don't worry, it is quite normal, and you won't do yourself or your baby any harm by being awake now and again, even for long spells of time. Do whatever feels right for you. You can rest in bed, or get up and do something to distract your mind. Learning to let go of your old "Eight hours a night" rigid sleep pattern is good preparation for when your baby arrives. There are many reasons why you might be struggling to sleep; you might be feeling uncomfortable, overly energetic, excited or simply worried. Think about ways to exercise and release some energy during the day and if you are worried or uncomfortable, try using a relaxation CD as these help switch off the part of your brain that is causing you stress and activate the part of your brain that makes you feel restful.'

Mood swings

Caught yourself sobbing at a cat food advert? Can't work out why you keep snapping at your partner for the littlest things? Blame those pregnancy hormones (again). Thanks to them, your moods become heightened and even minor events can send you from extremes of happiness to end-of-the-world doom and gloom.

But it's not just a chemical reaction. Thoughts about the future can also cause mood swings and worry. You may ask yourself 'Will I be a good mother?' 'Will I be able to cope during the birth?' 'How will motherhood affect my career?' Talk to somebody – whether it's your partner, mum, friend or midwife, it's very important to speak about how you're feeling.

REAL LIFE

'I felt premenstrual all the time!'

'Throughout my pregnancy I felt I was on an emotional rollercoaster. One minute I was on a complete high about becoming a mum, the next minute I was sobbing because I burnt the toast. My partner usually stayed out of my way when I was "having a moment".'

JODI, MUM TO FREDDIE, TWO
AND PEARL, THREE MONTHS

LIBIDO

There's a common misconception that pregnancy equals an end to sex (been there, done it, got the bump to prove it), but this isn't always the case. Some women find that pregnancy actually boosts their sexual appetite. A brilliant side effect of all the extra blood pumping around in pregnancy is that it creates heightened sensitivity in the clitoral area, which can lead to better or even multiple orgasms. Add to this the increase in hormones and not having to worry about contraception and you could be having some pretty satisfying sex right now. And pregnancy also signals a boost in your curves, which many partners can't get enough of.

Of course, pregnancy libido can go in the other direction. If you've been feeling exhausted, drained from nausea and sickness or just unsure about the many changes going on in your body, sex can be the last thing on your mind. However, you can still feel close to your partner. Less sex means more cuddles, which can still build intimacy. Non-sexual touching is important in any relationship, so take time for regular cuddles and kisses. Don't worry about the safety of sex during pregnancy. Unless you've been told by your doctor or midwife to refrain, it's perfectly safe and can't hurt your baby. For more tips on sex in pregnancy, see page 88.

EXTERNAL SYMPTOMS AND SIDE EFFECTS

While everything is going on inside you, you may also notice certain changes happening on the outside. From spots and blemishes to swollen ankles and even excess hair, it's all part of the joys of pregnancy. Many of these effects will be far more visible to you than anyone else, so try not to be paranoid and enjoy your pregnancy.

Q&A

'I've heard diet can help to reduce swelling during pregnancy. What foods should I be eating?'

Nutritionist **CHARLOTTE STIRLING-REED** says, 'There is minimal research around specific foods that help kidney function and reduce swelling, so I would focus on other ways to reduce swelling. Drink cold drinks to keep cool as hot weather can increase swelling. Make sure you get plenty of rest and avoid processed foods and other foods high in salt as this can increase fluid retention and therefore exacerbate the swelling. Lastly, try to eat healthily and eat your five fruit and vegetables a day, which will help to make sure you're getting plenty of nutrients and antioxidants to look after your kidneys and your immune system.'

Swelling

While you are pregnant, your body contains far more fluid than normal – for example your blood volume gradually increases by 40 to 50 per cent. Fluid tends to collect in the lowest parts of the body – the feet and ankles, causing the dreaded swollen ankles. But you may also notice swelling in the hands, fingers or wrists. If your swelling is very severe, you have stomach pain or headaches, and it comes on suddenly, it could be a sign of pre-eclampsia, a serious condition that can affect your baby. See your family doctor straight away.

Most swelling disappears after the birth, but in the meantime, there are steps you can take. Sit with your feet up where you can and wear loose clothing that isn't tight round the ankle. See if you can persuade your partner to give you a foot rub in the evening as that will help relieve some of the pressure. Gentle exercise can help to relieve swollen ankles, in particular, try rotating your foot five times in both directions to encourage blood to move back up the leg.

Spots and acne (again)

If you thought you'd left your teenage skin problems behind, you may be surprised by the appearance of spots and acne during pregnancy. Much like the affect of your hormones on your skin in your adolescent years, pregnancy hormones can

DID YOU KNOW?

Melasma (also known as chloasma) is skin pigmentation that can appear in pregnancy. It's sometimes known as the 'mask of pregnancy', because it appears on your face.

affect it too. But it can be upsetting when you were expecting the traditional pregnancy 'glow' and instead get pimples.

Make sure you eat plenty of fruits and vegetables and drink lots of water as that will improve the condition of the skin. Use a gentle cleanser – if it's too harsh it will strip the natural oils away, encouraging your skin to produce even more oil, which makes spots more likely. Moisturize with a light cream and avoid wearing heavy make-up if you can. Mineral-based powders are a good option. Your skin will calm down once your hormones return to normal after birth.

Varicose veins

Veins contain valves that keep blood flowing back towards the heart. If the valves fail you may notice bulging or varicose veins on your legs as the blood 'pools' behind the valves. The veins can also feel itchy, and they may throb and ache. People who suffer from varicose veins tend to already have a predisposition – often hereditary – but certain factors can increase the risk of developing them including pregnancy.

The weight of your baby, especially in the last trimester, presses on veins in the pelvis and makes it more difficult for blood to pass back up them. Plus, pregnancy hormones weaken the valves in your veins making the vein walls more stretchy and so the valves more prone to failing.

If you develop varicose veins, talk to your doctor. You may need further treatment after the baby is born, but until then wear compression stockings to relieve the discomfort and try sitting with your legs raised to help blood flow back up your legs – although this tends to only provide temporary relief. Don't cross your legs either as this can exacerbate the problem.

Once you've had your baby, talk to your doctor about whether any further treatment will be

DID YOU KNOW?

If you've spotted a dark line that goes down your bump from just under your belly button, it's known as a linea nigra. It's caused by a hormone produced by your growing placenta, which stimulates cells in the skin to produce extra pigment, and creates a dark line. They can also cause your nipples to appear darker.

needed, as varicose veins don't generally disappear and may even become worse in future pregnancies. He or she may refer you to a specialist who may suggest removing the affected veins surgically.

Excess hair

If you've noticed that the hair on your head seems thicker and more lustrous and plentiful, there's a chance you've also noticed it on other areas. It's due to increased hormone levels during pregnancy, which limit the usual cycle of shedding and growing new hair (on your head and body). As your hormones change again after pregnancy, this usually disappears and a few months after the birth you may notice lots of hair falling out before the normal balance is restored.

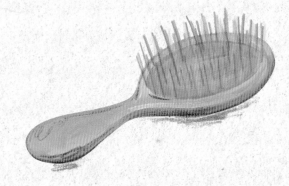

Stretch marks

As your bump (and other areas of your body) grows in size, you may notice red lines developing on the skin. Known as 'stretch marks' these affect about 80 per cent of women during pregnancy. You may have already developed the marks as they can also occur during rapid growth spurts or weight gain. They appear when outer layers of the skin, the epidermis, tear. You have them for life, but they'll fade to silvery white (if you're Caucasian) or yellow (if you have darker skin).

Stretch marks tend to run in families so if your own mum got them during pregnancy, the chances of you developing them are higher. They can make your skin feel itchy and dry, and massaging plenty of moisturizers or body oils into you skin will help soothe the irritation, but it won't stop stretch marks appearing. If you rub cream and oils in after the birth it will help them to fade, although won't make them disappear altogether .

However, if your skin is constantly itchy and this itching is accompanied by itchy palms and feet, it could be a sign of obstetric cholestasis, a potentially dangerous liver problem, so talk to your midwife or family doctor straight away.

UNEXPECTED SIDE EFFECTS

While you can expect pregnancy to cause aches and pains, you may also get some slightly more surprising side effects. In most cases, they're totally normal in their strangeness and all part and parcel of the crazy life of pregnancy.

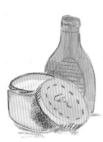

REAL LIFE

'My stretch marks remind me that I've got two amazing children'

'I noticed that I was developing stretch marks in my second pregnancy. I was so busy running around after my toddler and hadn't even thought about rubbing oils into my skin. They seemed quite red and angry-looking at first, but once Molly arrived, they were the least of my worries. They've now faded and while I can still see them, I don't mind them. They're a reminder that I've done this amazing thing: I carried two children and became a mother.'

CHRISSIE, MUM TO XANDER, FIVE,
AND MOLLY, 19 MONTHS

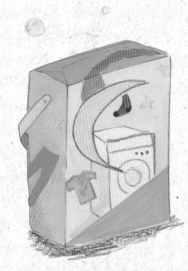

Cravings and pica

The jury is still out on what actually causes a pregnant woman to eat half a jar of pickles dipped in whipped cream or roast beef with strawberry jelly, but there's no doubt that pregnancy cravings are extremely common. There are generally two schools of thought about what causes cravings. One view is that they're your body's way of telling you you're deficient in a certain vitamin or mineral. The second is that it is caused by the changing hormones. Your levels of progesterone and oestrogen both fluctuate during pregnancy and at different times of day. A progesterone spike can make sweet things taste even better, while rising oestrogen can push you towards something saltier.

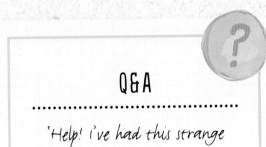

Q&A

'Help! I've had this strange desire to eat washing powder. What's causing it?'

GP **DR ELLIE CANNON** says, 'If you find yourself craving things that aren't edible, such as chalk, coal or soil, you're experiencing what's known as pica. We don't know why this can happen for some mums-to-be, but it's most likely linked to hormones. It definitely isn't wise or safe to give in to pica cravings, so talk to your family doctor or midwife if you're worried.'

Treat your cravings as you would any other part of your diet – if they're healthy, go for it, and if they're a bit more indulgent, enjoy in moderation. If you're having erratic or very intense hankerings, eating little and often may help settle them. This regulates your blood sugar levels, which in turn regulates your body's secretion of hormones. This results in fewer spikes, which could help you manage your cravings.

Your feet 'expand'

The hormone relaxin can cause ligaments in your feet to soften in pregnancy, leaving you more prone to sprains. Wear supportive footwear with a strap or laces such as trainers and, if you can, steer clear of flat ballet pumps and flip-flops (tough when you're pregnant during summer), as they'll provide no support for your feet. If you're wearing heels, pick ones that are 3cm (1in) or lower as any higher and you'll be off balance – especially with a growing bump.

It's also common for your feet to grow as the looser ligaments let your bones spread out a bit. It's nothing to worry about, but be warned, they may not return to their original size even after having your baby.

Susceptible to nosebleeds

Along with stuffiness (see page 29), pregnancy can leave you prone to nose bleeds. Hormonal changes soften the capillaries in your nose, making them more likely to rupture and bleed. You may find it's worse in cold weather because central heating leaves the mucous membranes in your nose irritated. Staying hydrated is key here. Prevent the lining of your nose from becoming too dry by using saline sprays and make sure you drink plenty of fluids; if the nose is moist it means fewer nosebleeds.

Bleeding gums

Don't panic if your gums bleed more than usual at the moment. Hormonal changes mean gums can become more swollen and bleed easily. You should still continue to brush and floss your teeth as normal, but if you're worried, use a soft bristled or electric toothbrush as these put less pressure on sensitive gums. If you are concerned go to your dentist for a checkup; remember, you get free dental care when you're pregnant and for a year after your baby's birth, so make the most of it.

Heightened sense of smell

You may have noticed that since becoming pregnant, you've become super-sensitive to smells and they seem much stronger than before. Food smells seem stronger and you can even smell other people where you would never have noticed their scent before (meaning your daily cramped train ride pushed up against a random man's armpit is even worse now you're pregnant). Nobody has really got to the bottom of what causes this heightened olfactory ability, but if you find that it is really affecting you, you can encourage your partner or friends to take over the cooking (if that's what's causing problems), avoid foods that make you feel unwell and also try carrying a handkerchief or tissue impregnanted with a gentle scent that you can endure so you can cover your nose and mask any unpleasant odours that are out of your control.

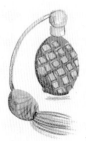

REAL LIFE

'Perfumes turned my stomach'

'When I was pregnant, I really noticed strong-smelling perfumes. Sometimes the smell would be so strong I'd feel a little light-headed and have to leave the room. I felt bad telling people that their favourite perfume was making me feel ill, but just had to explain that it was a side effect of pregnancy.'

MEGAN, MUM TO JOSEPH, THREE

DID YOU KNOW?

Pregnancy hormones influence the olfactory system – our sense of smell – so that smells and taste can seem stronger. It's thought this is so mums-to-be are more aware of foods that could potentially cause harm to her own health or that of her baby.

RED FLAG SYMPTOMS AND SIGNS

With any luck, your pregnancy will pass without a hitch, but it's worth being aware of red flag symptoms that could suggest there is something wrong. Dr Ellie Cannon reveals the ones you should be aware of. If you notice any of the following at any stage during your pregancy, call your doctor or midwife straight away.

Bleeding

If you start to get any kind of bleeding, it's vital to call your doctor even if the bleeding stops. In the early weeks of pregnancy, a little spotting or bleeding is very common, however, it could also be a sign of miscarriage. If you are in severe pain it could be an ectopic pregnancy, which is potentially life-threatening. Bleeding in the second or third trimesters may signal a problem with the mother or baby, for example, there may be something wrong with the placenta. Likewise, if you start leaking clear fluid with blood in it, it could mean your waters have broken and you've gone into labour. Call your doctor or midwife immediately.

Early labour

Any stomach pains or strong lower back pains could be contractions so keep an eye on them, especially if it's before 37 weeks. While you can get Braxton Hicks contractions (which are like practice contractions), and backache during pregnancy, if the pain is coming in regular intervals and increasing in frequency, it could be sign of early labour. If in doubt, speak to your midwife or doctor to get yourself checked out.

Vomiting, diarrhoea, fever or chills

These can be signs of an infection, so it's important to get yourself and your baby checked out to make sure it isn't something that could harm your baby if left untreated. This is particularly the case if you've been very sick and are having trouble keeping fluids down as you need to ensure you and your baby stay well hydrated.

Changes in vision

If you experience blurred or double vision, flashing spots or dimmed eyesight in the second half of your pregnancy this can be a sign of gestational diabetes (diabetes that can develop during pregnancy) or a potentially life-threatening condition called pre-eclampsia. Always talk to your doctor or midwife.

Frequent, painful headaches

Headaches can be caused by hormonal changes and the increase in blood circulating through your body. However, in the second half of pregnancy they can also be a symptom of pre-eclampsia. If your headaches are accompanied by vomiting, you should see a medical professional as soon as possible.

Decrease in your baby's movements

You'll probably start noticing obvious movements from your baby from when you're around 20 weeks pregnant, but they'll be quite faint. As your baby grows, the movements will become more obvious and you'll notice when he moves more or less. If you spot a difference in his movements, or your baby hasn't moved for a long time, have something sugary to eat or drink, and lie down and relax. Movements should start to happen pretty soon. If they don't, call your midwife as soon as possible.

Feelings of extreme sadness or depression

You have probably heard of postnatal depression, but prenatal depression can also occur in any pregnant woman. It is more common if you have a history of depression already. Look out for feelings of anxiety, helplessness, restlessness, lack of concentration, extreme insomnia and a loss of appetite. Always talk to your doctor or midwife if you've been feeling very low during pregnancy.

THE FIRST TRIMESTER

MONTH ONE

Doctors count the beginning of your pregnancy as the first day of your last period so, strange as it seems, you might not even be pregnant for around the first two weeks of your pregnancy.

The beginning of week 5 is when your next period would be due. This is when most women suspect they're pregnant and do a pregnancy test.

WEEK 5

MONTH 1

MONTH 2

WEEK 2

WEEK 1

Your pregnancy is dated from the first day of your last period...

WEEK 3

...although conception occurs days after intercourse, between weeks 2 and 3.

WEEK 4

Your fertilized egg is now separating into an embryo and a placenta.

BABY SIZE: SESAME SEED

Your baby's eyes and earlobes are now formed but she won't open her eyes until week 27.

WEEK 9

WEEK 7

WEEK 8

WEEK 6

MONTH 3

MONTH THREE

Four out of five women are affected by morning sickness but it can happen at any time of day.

MONTH TWO

Most women are alerted to the possibility that they are pregnant when their period is late. The pregnancy test kits that you buy from chemists are extremely accurate, but they can give false negatives if your period is slightly irregular. If you are unsure, repeat the test a few days later; most kits contain two test sticks. If your test is positive, it's time to make an appointment with your doctor.

WEEK 10

Decide where to give birth. Now is the time to talk to your doctor about whether you want to have your baby in hospital, a midwife unit or at home.

WEEK 11

BABY SIZE: FIG

WEEK 12

It's your decision when to spread the happy news of your pregnancy, but consider telling a close work friend before others if you are suffering from morning sickness and exhaustion.

WEEK 13

The placenta is now fully formed and supplies your baby's food and oxygen.

NOTES

NOTES

....

CONGRATULATIONS — YOU'VE MADE
IT THROUGH THE FIRST EXCITING THREE
MONTHS OF YOUR PREGNANCY —
THE BEST IS YET TO COME!

....

CHAPTER SIX
SECOND TRIMESTER

Your second trimester (months four to six) is often one of the most exciting times of your pregnancy: you can finally tell people your news (so no more sneaky soda waters masquerading as a gin and tonic); your body is beginning to change shape; and and part way through you'll start to feel the first gentle movements of your baby. Plus, after the tiring fogginess of the first three months, you'll finally have a bit of energy, which means you may start feeling like doing fun things such as buying yourself some maternity clothes or signing up for pregnancy exercise classes.

MONTH FOUR

It can seem ironic that after the first few months of your pregnancy, when you knew you were pregnant (thanks to the frequent trips to the loo, the nausea, and the exhaustion) but few others did, just as you begin to let people know you're pregnant many of these symptoms will begin to disappear. The lack of discernible bump at this stage leaves some women wondering if there's really a baby in there. Rest assured, you'll gradually start noticing changes to your body over the next few weeks. If it helps, try downloading an app that tells you what size your baby is at each stage, and how he's developing so you can visualize him inside you.

Your body begins to change

Ok, so the bump still has some way to go, but it's about now that you may start to notice a bit of a curve on your stomach (although it may still resemble a big lunch belly). At this stage, your baby weighs about 23g (less than 1oz) and is approximately 7cm (2¾in)long – about the size of a small chocolate bar. The reproductive organs are already developing. A boy's testes will be formed and his penis will be inside his body. A baby girl will already have fully formed ovaries containing two million eggs. However, it's probably still too early to tell what the gender is from an ultrasound – you can usually find this out at your 20-week anomaly scan if you want to.

Taking exercise

With any luck, morning sickness has abated, your energy levels have improved and you're feeling ready for some exercise.

If you took regular exercise before you got pregnant, you may be able to continue as before, just ensuring you've made a few changes to allow for your condition. If you attend a class tell the instructor that you're pregnant or if you're

a member of a gym, talk to a member of staff to tell them. Your instructor or one of the personal trainers at the gym should be able to give you some pointers on how you should adapt your workout, or whether you need to change the class.

Other great activities to take up include yoga for pregnancy, swimming and walking. Turn to page 76 to find out what to bear in mind when doing these exercises and how you can maintain an active lifestyle right up to your due date.

MONTH FIVE

Congratulations, you've reached the halfway mark. You'll definitely notice your growing bump as your baby continues to develop. In fact, he'll be growing so fast now that his weight will double over the next month and will overtake the weight of the placenta. Your baby will be covered in fine downy hair called lanugo, which helps to regulate his temperature, and a greasy substance called vernix forms a waterproof barrier on his skin (this will probably still be on his skin when he is born). He will show up more clearly on an ultrasound scan because he's starting to lay down more calcium in his bones. Make sure you get plenty of calcium-rich foods such as dairy products in your diet to help with this. Your baby will take all the calcium he needs from you, leaving you short if you don't keep your levels topped up.

You'll also have had your second antenatal check-up by this point (you'll have 10 in total throughout your pregnancy if you're a first-time mum). But one of the most exciting and nerve-wracking moments is having your 20-week anomaly scan (see opposite).

Weight gain

While it's not the best time to be obsessing about weight, you should be aware of your weight and how it's fluctuating throughout your pregnancy. It is important to maintain a healthy diet. You don't need a special diet nor do you need to eat for two (see right).

Your midwife will check your weight at your antenatal appointments, mainly so that she can keep track of whether you're becoming overweight, which can bring with it a risk of gestational diabetes.

Confirmation of your pregnancy

You will probably have told your workplace that you're pregnant by now – once they know you can take paid time off for antenatal appointments. From 20 weeks, your midwife should give you a certificate of pregnancy – the MAT B1 form – to give to your employer or take to the social services department if you are not working. This entitles you to take your maternity leave and get maternity pay. Sign the form and give it to your employer before you are 25 weeks pregnant (by the end of the 15th week before the beginning of your expected week of birth). Now's the time to let your employers know your due date in writing and when you think you'll want to start your maternity leave.

EXPERT TIP

MANAGING WEIGHT GAIN

If you're a normal weight, you'll probably find you put on about 10–12 kg (1½–1¾ stone) during your pregnancy but this changes if you were underweight or overweight to begin with. Some women lose weight in their first trimester due to morning sickness or simply because their pregnancy has encouraged them to reassess their eating habits. Remember, it's not just your bump that is growing in size. You'll also be laying down fat in your bottom, hips and thighs, to help fuel breastfeeding once your baby is born. Your breasts will also be increasing in size as the milk ducts develop.

Dr Ellie Cannon
GP

DID YOU KNOW?

Eating for two is a myth (sorry)! You need just 200 extra calories on top of the usual 2,000 calories when you're pregnant, but only in the final trimester.

THE 20-WEEK ANOMALY SCAN

Halfway through your pregnancy (or realistically sometime between weeks 18–22), you'll have a second scan, which is known as your anomaly scan.

This gives you a more advanced picture of your baby and checks he's growing at the correct rate. The sonographer will take measurements of his head, abdomen and thigh bones and look at his face for a cleft palate (when the top of the mouth and lip doesn't form properly) and his spine for defects such as spina bifida. They will check your baby's heart to make sure blood is flowing through it correctly and examine other organs such as the stomach, kidneys and bladder to make sure there are no abnormalities. He or she will also examine your uterus and placenta . The position of the placenta will be observed to ensure it is not lying too close to the cervix. Blood flow through the umbilical cord will be assessed and he or she will check that that you have enough amniotic fluid.

You can usually find out the gender of your baby at this scan. A skilled sonographer can pick out your baby's sex organs on an ultrasound, so if you don't want to know, make sure you tell him or her.

QUICK FIX

DECODE YOUR SCAN NOTES

AC: Abdominal circumference

BPD: Biparietal diameter – the measurement from one side of your baby's head to the other – ear to ear

OFD: Occipitofrontal diameter – the front-to-back measurement of his head

CRL: Crown-to-rump length. The length from the top of your baby's head to his bottom

HC: Head circumference

FL: Femoral length – the length of your baby's thigh bone

GA: Gestational age, or the age of your baby in the womb

EDD: Estimated date of delivery – your 'due date'

EFW: Estimated foetal weight – how much the sonographer thinks your baby will weigh at birth

Q&A

'At my 20-week scan, my sonographer said I had a low-lying placenta. Will I need a Caesarean?'

Midwife **HELEN TAYLOR** says, 'A placenta that is near, or partially or totally covers the cervix can pose a risk to you both as the baby's exit route may be obstructed. The good news is as your uterus grows with advancing pregnancy, it often pulls the placenta up out of the way so you will be given another scan closer to your due date. If the placenta is still covering the cervix, you are likely to need a Caesarean delivery. In the meantime call your doctor or midwife if there's any bleeding.'

MONTH SIX

You're now over half way through your pregnancy, and you will be preparing yourself and your home for your baby's arrival. You'll probably be looking into the different pieces of kit you'll need once your baby arrives, including a car seat, pram and/or buggy, Moses basket and a cot.

Meanwhile, your baby is still growing and developing. He'll have started practising various movements that will be vital for him after birth, including those needed for breathing. He won't actually be breathing as he gets all the oxygen he needs from the blood supply coming from your placenta, and the air sacs in his lungs are full of a product called surfactant that stops them from collapsing.

You will feel movements much more obviously now. Your baby will be beginning to get into a pattern of sleeping and waking, but it won't necessarily coincide with yours. You might be in bed, feeling relaxed and ready for sleep while your baby is wide awake and moving about.

ANTENATAL CLASSES

Now's the time to start thinking about antenatal classes. There's a massive selection out there – some are free, some you pay for. Different classes offer different types of support: some focus on pregnancy, birth and child care, others are exercise-based, or concentrate on specific birth methods. What is important is to book yourself in early – especially for the free ones – as spaces fill up quickly. The classes usually run for three to six weeks, often in the evenings, although some take place over the weekend. Ask your doctor or midwife or check the internet to see what is available in your area.

Specialist organizations such as the National Childbirth Trust (NCT) run classes. These are often small groups, and usually go into more detail than those run by the health service and may have a stronger focus on the emotional side of pregnancy and birth. The intimacy of the classes means you're likely to forge strong bonds with your fellow mums-to-be. Plus, because they're local, it means that all the mums in it will live nearby, which is useful for pre- and post-baby coffee mornings. Prices vary depending on where you live and the type of class.

If you want advice in your classes for specific birth methods, such as hypnobirthing or active birth ask your midwife or look on the internet. Find out how much of the technical side of birth they cover and whether you'll need a top up of information from a regular class.

Try a maternity retreat

Fancy indulging in spa treatments and gourmet food alongside your classes? A weekend retreat could be for you. These are obviously the most expensive, but can be a nice way to combine some pre-baby pampering while learning about the birth at the same time.

START BONDING WITH YOUR BUMP

Maternal instinct doesn't appear as soon as the line appears on your pregnancy test. Luckily, you can arm yourself with strategies that will help you feel closer to your baby.

Rock on

Moving gently from side to side will help soothe your baby in the amniotic sac. Babies feel instinctively safer and secure when rocked (now and when they're born). Sit on the floor and rock in circles, or just try gentle swinging dance moves.

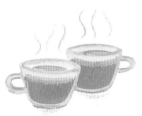

REAL LIFE

'Antenatal classes set me up with lifelong friends'

'When I was pregnant with my first baby, I signed up for national childbirth trust classes in my local area. They're not cheap, but I'd heard they're a great way to meet new mums in my area. The information provided in the classes was useful, but by far the best thing about them was that I now have a bunch of mum friends who live nearby, all with babies a similar age to mine. I've gone on to have a second child, as have many of the women in my class. Now all of our children play together while we provide support and company for each other. It's been wonderful to watch our children grow up together.'

CHARLIE, MUM TO ALICE, FOUR AND PETER, TWO

Take the plunge

Whether that's a dip at your local pool or a long relaxing bath, the sensation of being in water is soothing for you and your baby. Plus, exercise will trigger endorphins – happy hormones – that will cross the placenta, benefiting your baby, too.

Put pen to paper

Write a letter to your unborn baby or you could even start a diary. Write down how you feel, and try imagining what he will be like in the future and what your hopes and dreams are for him.

Have a chat

Talking to your tummy boosts your baby's ability to detect subtle differences in sounds after he's born, so he'll recognize the voices he's heard. Encourage your partner to talk to your bump as well; it's a great way for him to bond, too.

Picture your baby

Keep a copy of your scan picture in your wallet or bag to help you visualize your baby. This will help you kick start an emotional connection that will strengthen when you meet.

EXPERT TIP

GET SINGING

Say goodnight to your bump when you go to bed and sing him a short lullaby. Your baby will learn to love this song, and you can use it to soothe him after he's born too. I promise you, your baby will love your singing, even if everyone else thinks it is dreadful.

Mia Scotland
Doula

COPING AT WORK

Now that your workplace knows that you are pregnant, you can ensure you get all the rights and benefits offered to pregnant women.

If you work in an environment that isn't suitable for you now, such as a job with lots of lifting or where you need to be exposed to dangerous chemicals, your employer will need to find you alternative work that removes you from that situation. And if there is no alternative, you should be suspended on full pay for as long as necessary to avoid the risk.

Pregnant employees have four main rights:

- Paid time off for antenatal care
- Maternity leave
- Maternity pay or maternity allowance
- Protection against unfair treatment, discrimination or dismissal

It's worth noting that 'antenatal care' does not just mean medical appointments. You can have time off for antenatal or parenting classes if they've been recommended by your doctor or midwife.

Make sure you look after yourself at work. Take regular breaks including one for lunch. Make sure you stay hydrated, eat properly, and sit properly at your desk. You can ask your employer for a work place assessment to make sure that your desk and chair are set up correctly to prevent problems such as repetitive strain injuries (RSI) or back problems.

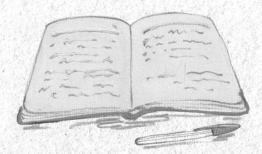

If you're struggling with pregnancy brain (and let's face it, who doesn't get it?), make lists. Write down what you hope to achieve each day (or the next day) at work, listing them in order of importance or deadline.

Start thinking about your maternity leave handover now. Whether or not you're involved in hiring the person who will cover your role, it's a good idea to start tying up any loose ends before you finish. You could also start putting together a handover document with information and advice now so you don't have to do it all in your last week when you're already tired and distracted.

TRAVELLING WHILE PREGNANT

Once your baby arrives, holidays are likely to take on a very different pattern to those of your pre-baby days so it's a good idea to book a babymoon together – a pre-baby holiday – before the birth.

Obviously, if you're pregnant, certain activities aren't suitable (you can rule out skiing, surfing and rock-climbing), but there are plenty of locations you can visit that are perfect for a relaxing long weekend. Hotels with spas are ideal, especially if you don't have to fly there because they'll be easier to get to – this is important in the later stages of your pregnancy (see below). Make use of the relaxing spa treatments to pamper yourself before your baby's arrival.

DID YOU KNOW?

Most airlines will not allow women who are 36 or more weeks pregnant to fly. Some will with a doctor's letter; check before booking a trip.

TRAVEL CHECKLIST

WHEN PLANNING A TRIP (EITHER AT HOME OR ABROAD) REMEMBER THE FOLLOWING:

- Take your maternity notes in case something happens and you need to see a doctor while away.

- Check that your medical insurance covers you while pregnant.

- Wear DVT socks if flying. You're at a higher risk of deep vein thrombosis during pregnancy because of the increased pressure on the veins in your legs and pelvis. Get up and walk around when you can.

- Check your holiday destination won't require you to have vaccinations, as they might not be suitable during pregnancy.

Car journeys with a bump

Whether it's a road trip or a quick journey to the shops, driving with a bump can be a challenge.

Having a big bump is no excuse to stop belting up in the car. Wear the lap portion so that it fits across your thighs and hips, and *under* your bump – not across it. Place the diagonal strap over your collarbone, then down between your breasts. Fasten it so that it sits *above* your bump, not on it.

If you're going on a long journey, make sure you take regular breaks to prevent your legs and ankles becoming swollen (just like you would if you were on a plane). Although you're likely to need to visit the loo regularly anyway. If you are prone to backache, wedge a cushion in the small of your back to help ease the discomfort.

CHAPTER SEVEN
DIET AND LIFESTYLE IN PREGNANCY

Pregnancy often encourages women to really look at their lifestyle, and in many cases, give it a complete overhaul. Suddenly, you're not just thinking about yourself, you also need to take the right steps to protect and nurture your growing baby's health, too. There are plenty of things you can do in your day-to-day life to ensure you have a healthy and safe pregnancy.

CONTINUE WITH SUPPLEMENTS

In an ideal world, we'd be able to get all our nutrients from our food or environment. The reality is a little different, and when it comes to pregnancy, opting for a supplement can ensure you get the vitamins and minerals you both need.

As long as you're having a healthy pregnancy, there are only two vitamins you're advised to take as a supplement: folic acid (one of the B vitamins) and vitamin D. You will hopefully have already been taking them while trying to conceive (see page 15), and it's worth continuing once you are pregnant. If you decide to take a general multi-vitamin avoid any that contain vitamin A (anything with cod liver oil for example) as too much vitamin A can cause kidney problems.

Folic acid

This nutrient is vital for the proper development of your baby's spinal cord, and it can protect against neural tube defects. A lack of it can lead to a condition known as spina bifida, which occurs when the protective covering around the baby's spinal cord doesn't form properly. This can lead to nerve damage and paralysis.

Your baby's spinal cord develops early in your pregnancy – within the first 12 weeks – which is why it's so important to take folic acid during your first trimester if not before. You can stop once you reach 13 weeks, but it also works with vitamin B12 to help in the formation of red blood cells, so you may want to continue. You'll need a daily supplement of 4mg, but you can also eat folate-rich foods such as spinach, broccoli, asparagus, eggs, brown rice and fortified cereals.

Vitamin D

This is another nutrient that pregnant women should take as a supplement. This is because the main source of vitamin D is the action of the sun on our skin. However, most of northern Europe, for example, doesn't often get enough sunlight for anyone to receive their daily requirement, especially during the winter months, so it's best to top up any levels you do have with a supplement. This is worse if you have dark skin or cover yourself up.

You should take a supplement containing 1mg of vitamin D to help in the absorption of calcium, which is needed by your baby to develop healthy bones and teeth.

Iron

This mineral is very important during pregnancy to make red blood cells (haemoglobin), which you'll have more of as the volume of blood in your body increases. However, despite the extra needs, the recommended daily amount of iron (14.8mg) does not increase when you are pregnant because you're not losing any blood through your period.

Even so, it's often during pregnancy that many women discover they are deficient in the nutrient (anaemic), and probably were before they got pregnant. However, the symptoms of anaemia – such as tiredness, fatigue and breathlessness – become more pronounced now. Also, your midwife will be keeping an eye on haemoglobin levels and take regular blood tests throughout your pregnancy so will be able to detect whether you are anaemic and provide you with iron pills.

DID YOU KNOW?

You can also find vitamin D in some foods, including oily fish, eggs, meat, fortified breakfast cereals and margarine.

Q&A

'I started taking folic acid at six weeks when I discovered I was pregnant. Is my baby in danger?'

Nutritionist **CHARLOTTE STIRLING-REED** says, 'The most important thing is to take it as soon as you realize you are pregnant. It is recommended that women take folic acid as a safeguard when they are trying for a baby. Mums should take it as early as possible if they are already pregnant.'

EXPERT TIP

IRON SUPPLEMENTS

If your doctor recommends you take an iron supplement, watch out for constipation, which can be a common side effect. Opt for plenty of fruits, vegetables and wholemeal carbohydrates to help boost your fibre intake. The fruits and vegetables may also contain vitamin C, which helps to aid the absorption of iron.

Charlotte Stirling-Reed
Nutritionist

YOUR PREGNANCY DIET

Right now your body is doing the amazing job of growing your baby, so it's essential you nourish it well so you can fuel his development and boost your energy levels. Eating well in pregnancy means having a normal, healthy diet – although there some foods you should avoid (see pages 68–9). You may feel hungrier, but this is often because you're tired and craving foods that give you energy – it does not mean you should eat more than usual.

A diet that incorporates low glycaemic index (low GI) foods that release energy slowly will help to maintain even blood sugar levels, and prevent the dips and highs that can have you reaching for the nearest chocolate bar. Keeping sugar levels on an even keel will maintain your energy levels and stop your feeling too hungry.

Ideally, you should eat a healthy balance of carbohydrates, protein and fats, with plenty of vitamin- and mineral-rich foods. Of course, the reality can be very different. If you're suffering from sickness and nausea in your first trimester, you may struggle to keep much food down and the food that does stay put is more likely to be crisps and dry toast.

The good news is that whatever you eat your baby will take all the nutrients he needs. You can maintain your energy and aid his development by eating the right balance of carbohydrates, protein, dairy, fats, fruit and vegetables.

Carbohydrates

These are vital in pregnancy as they provide much-needed energy. Think potatoes, bread, rice and pasta, but where you can, pick the wholemeal or whole grain varieties of these foods. They usually have a low or medium glycaemic-index rating and they will boost your fibre intake, which is useful during pregnancy when digestion can get a little sluggish. Aim to eat a portion of carbohydrates with every meal.

Protein

Foods rich in protein help to build your baby's cells and tissues and they'll repair yours. Aim for two or three portions a day. Meat, eggs, cheese, seeds, cereals, soya and pulses are all great sources of protein. Fish is also packed with protein, but limit oily fish (salmon, fresh tuna, mackerel, trout and sardines) to no more than two portions a week, because they can contain pollutants such as dioxins and PCBs (polychlorinated biphenyls) and tuna contains some mercury. Also avoid swordfish and shark as they contain mercury pollutants (see pages 68–9).

Dairy

It's vital to provide your baby with calcium for bone development, so aim for two or three portions of dairy products a day. Your baby's bones will be prioritized when it comes to getting enough calcium, so if you don't eat enough your bones and teeth may be weakened. Hard cheese, yogurt and milk are great sources of calcium. Drink semi-skimmed milk rather than skimmed milk as it also contains vitamins A, D, E and K and essential fats. If you don't eat dairy, you can find similar nutrients in watercress, spinach, broccoli and almonds, and in enriched soya and rice milks.

Fats

Often considered the least healthy area of a diet, they are necessary, so don't cut them out; just pick the right ones. Fats help with the hormonal regulation of your energy levels, and essential fats (the ones found in oily fish, flaxseed oil, seeds, nuts and avocado) are vital for your baby's brain and spinal development. Watch out for unhealthy transfats found in processed foods.

Fruits and vegetables

Get your five-a-day fruit and vegetables and you're on the right track. Make sure each portion is different (so three apples and two bananas doesn't count) and try to eat a rainbow of colours as the variety will provide the richest array of nutrients. Green leafy vegetables such as spinach or cabbage are great sources of vitamins B and C, needed for energy and a healthy immune system, while brightly coloured foods such as aubergines, peppers and tomatoes are rich in antioxidants, needed for healthy functioning in your body. Make sure you wash all fruit and vegetables before eating or cooking to remove traces of soil.

Q&A

'I'm a vegetarian – how can I make sure I get all the nutrients I need during pregnancy?'

Nutritionist **CHARLOTTE STIRLING-REED** says, 'The most important thing to do is eat a variety of foods every day – this will make sure you get all the nutrients you and your growing baby need. Make sure you include foods such as pulses, nuts and seeds or even meat alternatives such as Quorn and tofu to ensure you have nutrients found in meat products such as iron and B vitamins. Eating foods high in vitamin C such as citrus fruits, dark green leafy vegetables and peppers with a meal can also help your body absorb more of the iron.'

YOUR NEW FOOD RULES

When it comes to foods you should be avoiding in pregnancy, this is a little more complicated. While there are certain foods that are a definite no-go area, there are some exceptions to the rule. Vitamin A is stored in the liver and high doses can cause birth defects and liver toxicity, so avoid multi-vitamins that contain it. Preformed vitamin A (used directly by the body) is found in animal products like eggs, milk, and liver so you should limit your intake of these foods, but you can eat as many carotenoids (which the body converts into vitamin A) as you want. In addition, if there's a family history of food allergies, for example to nuts, avoid these foods in pregnancy.

If you are a vegetarian or vegan

If you don't eat animal products, a healthy diet is especially important. Vegetarians should ensure they get enough iron and include both varieties – haem (from animal products) and non-haem. You may need to take a haem iron supplement and non-haem is found in fruits and vegetables. Vitamin B12 is another important nutrient largely found in animal products, but it's also in fortified breakfast cereals, yeast extract and soya products.

If you're vegan, as well as ensuring you get enough iron and vitamin B12, make sure you're getting enough calcium as it's needed for healthy bones and teeth. Your baby will take all the calcium he needs from you, so you need to top up your own levels to ensure good bone and dental health. Broccoli, kale, cabbage, almonds, sesame seeds, tahini, dates and tofu are all good sources. If you think that you might be missing certain nutrients talk to your midwife about supplements.

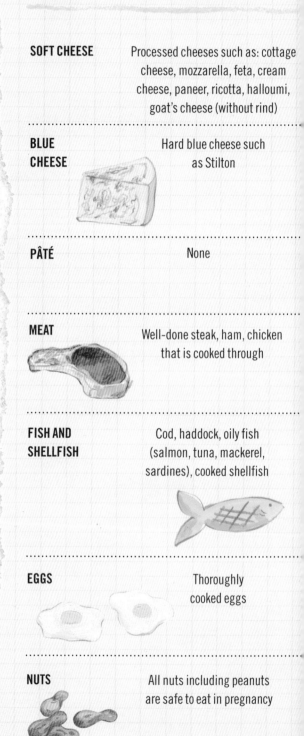

FOOD	CAN EAT
SOFT CHEESE	Processed cheeses such as: cottage cheese, mozzarella, feta, cream cheese, paneer, ricotta, halloumi, goat's cheese (without rind)
BLUE CHEESE	Hard blue cheese such as Stilton
PÂTÉ	None
MEAT	Well-done steak, ham, chicken that is cooked through
FISH AND SHELLFISH	Cod, haddock, oily fish (salmon, tuna, mackerel, sardines), cooked shellfish
EGGS	Thoroughly cooked eggs
NUTS	All nuts including peanuts are safe to eat in pregnancy

DON'T EAT	REASON	EXCEPTIONS TO THE RULE
Mould-ripened cheeses such as Brie or Camembert	Some soft cheeses can contain listeria, which can cause listeriosis, which can harm your unborn baby	You can eat Brie or Camembert if it's baked until it's piping hot all the way through. Don't eat any soft cheese made from unpasteurized milk
Soft blue cheses such as Roquefort, Danish blue, cambozola, Gorgonzola	Uncooked blue cheeses contain a mould (hence the colour) and have a high moisture content, so carry the risk of listeria. Hard cheeses contain less moisture, which reduces the risk	Cooked soft blue cheese (in a sauce for example) is safe to eat. Don't eat any hard blue cheese made from unpasteurized milk
Meat (especially liver) or vegetable pâté	All pâté carries a risk of listeria, and liver pâté contains dangerous levels of vitamin A as it is stored in the liver	
Undercooked meats (for example, pink steak or chicken), cured meat such as salami	Uncooked meat carries a risk of food poisoning, which can be dangerous for your baby	Cured meats such as chorizo or salami are safe to eat if cooked (on a pizza for example)
Swordfish, marlin, shark and raw shellfish	Limit portions of oily fish to two portions a week (see page 67). Raw shellfish carries a food poisoning risk, while swordfish, marlin and shark all contain high levels of mercury	Raw fish in sushi is safe if it has been frozen to -20°C (-4°F) beforehand (most commercially sold sushi is) as this kills the potentially dangerous parasitic worm. Although smoked salmon isn't cooked, the smoking process kills any bacteria
Raw eggs	Raw eggs can pose a salmonella risk, so look out for dishes where they might appear including home-made mayonnaise and mousses	
Don't eat nuts if there is a family history of nut allergy	Food allergies are often hereditary	

DRINKS IN PREGNANCY

When it comes to drinks in pregnancy, it's important that you make some adjustments. Certain drinks are more or less off the menu, while others need to be limited for the safety of your growing baby. Luckily, that doesn't mean there aren't plenty of choices out there for you.

It's also extremely important that you stay hydrated in pregnancy. Fluids not only make sure the normal cell processes within the body happen, but they are needed to ensure there are enough fluids for the baby, including amniotic fluid.

Limit caffeine

If you can't get through the first few hours of the day without your morning cup of coffee, you can still enjoy it, you'll just need to make sure you limit it to 200mg of caffeine each day. This is the equivalent of two cups of instant coffee or one cup of brewed coffee. However, if you enjoy coffee from chain outlets, bear in mind the caffeine content of their espresso-based drinks can vary massively; many automatically add a 'double shot' to these drinks. Check before you order.

Remember, 200mg is your total caffiene allowance for the day. If you drink tea or green tea, the caffeine content should be accounted for. A cup of regular black tea contains 75mg caffeine and a cup of green tea contains 50mg. Don't forget cola or caffeinated energy drinks; colas contain about 40mg and an energy drink contains 80mg (and sometimes more). It might be worth swapping your regular coffee, tea or cola for a decaffeinated version, as you often can't tell the difference in the flavour.

Caffeine is bad in pregnancy as it can cross the placenta and affect your baby in the same way as you; he may seem more fidgety after you've had your morning coffee. Studies have also shown that excess caffeine increases your risk of having a low birth weight baby. This in turn means that your baby is more likely to develop diabetes, high blood pressure and heart disease in later life.

Avoid alcohol

Current guidance states you should avoid alcohol throughout pregnancy, especially in the first three months. If you do choose to drink then keep it to 1-2 units once or twice a week – that's a small (175ml/6floz) glass of wine or 568ml (1 pint) of lager. However, it's important you check the alcohol percentage when ordering drinks, as some drinks have a higher alcohol content, which would mean the same volume of drink would actually be more units. This is especially the case with strong lagers and ciders.

Alcohol can pass through the placenta and enter your baby's blood stream and an unborn

EXPERT TIP

....

STRUGGLING WITH NAUSEA?

Some people find ginger helps. Make up a refreshing iced version of ginger tea by adding boiling water to freshly grated ginger. Leave it to cool for a few minutes, then add plenty of ice and serve in a tall glass.

Charlotte Stirling-Reed
Nutritionist

baby's immature liver can't break down alcohol as fast as yours can. So if you drink more than the recommended maximum amount of alcohol your baby is exposed to greater levels of alcohol than you, and for longer.

Constant excesive drinking in pregnancy can even lead to foetal alcohol syndrome (FAS). This condition results in babies with heart and kidney problems, and abnormal facial features such as a small head, a flat face, narrow eye slits and a loss of the groove between the nose and lips. Children with FAS also tend to be hyperactive, unable to concentrate and have poor social skills.

Luckily, there are plenty of other options for when those around you are drinking and you want to feel involved. If everyone's tucking into fizz, try some sparkling grape juice, make up your own mocktails using different fruit juices or simply have a glass of soda water and freshly squeezed lime. Apart from anything else, you'll save plenty of money while on the pregnancy drinking wagon.

Healthy drink options

Natural herbal teas are good during pregnancy as they're decaffeinated. Go for ginger in the first trimester if morning sickness is an issue, peppermint to help digestion and chamomile at night to help you relax and sleep. Another good drink for the first trimester and during labour is coconut water. It's naturally rich in electrolytes, minerals that help the body stay hydrated. Coconut water is great if you've been suffering from nausea or diarrhoea, sweating a lot or working hard during labour and need to replace lost fluids.

For a natural energy boost during pregnancy, choose a vegetable juice or smoothie over a fruit juice. This is because there are fewer sugars in vegetables, so they're less likely to give you the

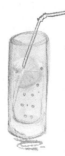

REAL LIFE

'I planned work drinks carefully'

'My job has a big after-work drinks culture, so when I found out I was pregnant, I dreaded them, especially in the first trimester when I wasn't ready to tell anyone. I made sure I knew what bar we'd be visiting in the evening and drop in a few hours before to explain the situation so they could "play along". I would always try and go to the same bartender, and when I asked for a gin and tonic, he would give me a plain tonic water and lime. I did it with all the bars near my office and it worked perfectly.'

VANESSA, 23 WEEKS PREGNANT

sugar high and subsequent slump that you can get after a strawberry and banana smoothie. Try making a vegetable smoothie with avocado – it's rich in healthy fats, is naturally sweet and has a smooth creamy texture. Add in kale (rich in calcium), cucumber for flavour and chia seeds (rich in omega-3 fatty acids) and you've got the perfect energy-boosting shake.

KEEPING CALM

Finding out you're pregnant can be exciting, but it can also raise a lot of worries or leave you feeling stressed. You may be concerned about how you'll cope as a mum, how to prepare yourself for the birth or you may simply be rushing around trying to get everything done before your baby arrives. It is important to make time for yourself to relax and de-stress. How you do this can vary from person to person. Some find it helps to have a warm bath or a cuddle from their partner. Others enjoy watching their favourite DVD box-set or picking out items for their baby. The benefits are that these give you some much-needed 'me time'.

However, there are also specific methods and practices that can help to keep you calm, and get you in the right frame of mind to be ready for this new chapter in your life. They can even help you stay relaxed during labour.

Mindfulness

If you spend your whole time thinking ahead and worrying about what's going to happen in the next week, month or even years, it can leave you feeling overwhelmed. That's where mindfulness comes in. It encourages you to put yourself in the moment and focus on what's around you right now. This blocks any future worries and helps you to relax. It could be something as simple as focusing on your surroundings as you walk to work – the sights and smells, the feel of the wind (or rain) on your face, and taking it all in. It will make a change from hurrying to work with your head down and your mind worrying about the emails or deadlines you have to meet. Mindfulness helps you become more aware of how your mind works, so instead of being overwhelmed by your thoughts you learn to manage them.

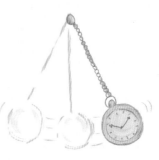

REAL LIFE

'I felt calm and in control thanks to a hypnobirthing course'

'I did a five-week course of two-hour lessons, which also included a book and CD. I learnt breathing and self-hypnosis exercises and massage techniques as well, and how a combination of these can help you overcome any fears. We were also taught optimal birth positions and the role your birth partner can play in labour. The course left me feeling very calm and in control as my due date approached and I was even sleeping better. When my surges, or contractions, began my partner and I practiced the relaxation techniques for about five hours. We then went into hospital where the midwife found that I was already 5cm (2in) dilated. I stayed focused throughout and just let my body take over. The midwives couldn't believe how calm I was. I managed to deliver Josephine naturally with no pain relief.'

CLAUDIA, MUM TO JOSEPHINE,
EIGHT MONTHS

Visualization

If you've ever noticed how reminiscing about your amazing beach holiday helps you feel calmer and happier, you'll understand the idea behind visualization as a means of relaxation. The practice is used by people in all walks of life, including top athletes, who use it to help them achieve their sporting goals. In pregnancy it's great for keeping you calm and often forms parts of other relaxation techniques including hypnobirthing (see below).

It can be useful if you're feeling overwhelmed or stressed about a particular issue of pregnancy or birth. But it can also be used if you're struggling to sleep or just need some time to yourself.

Hypnotherapy

While you can use hypnotherapy at any point in your life, it is especially useful during pregnancy as it can be used to help you through labour as well as keep you relaxed in the run up to the birth. The idea behind hypnotherapy for pregnancy and birth – or hypnobirthing as it is sometimes known – is that you put yourself in control of your labour and approach it with a different attitude. You use a different language, so rather than saying you're having a painful contraction, it's described as a 'tightening' or 'surge'. Rather than saying you have to push yourself through labour, you 'breathe' through it.

It is important to reduce fear and tension so that your labour can progress well. Famous obstetrician and pregnancy and birth expert Dr Grantly Dick-Read first introduced the idea of a fear-tension-pain cycle saying that a tense mind means a tense cervix. Studies have found hypnobirthing can reduce the need for pain relief drugs, increases the chance of a vaginal birth without assisted delivery and improves overall satisfaction and maternal wellbeing.

EXPERT TIP

TRY VISUALIZATION

This stimulates relaxation hormones. Get comfortable and turn your phone off. Take two long deep breaths, close your eyes, and picture yourself in your favourite place in nature – on a beach or in a forest or a meadow. Experiment to find the one that works for you. Lose yourself by focusing on what you can see, hear, smell and feel. Imagine the colours, the views around you, maybe there are people, trees or horizons? Listen to the birdsong or the sound of waves on the beach. Feel the sun on your face, the water at your toes. You could also imagine yourself in this place while holding your baby in your arms. Feel the weight of your baby, look into her eyes, and be aware of them looking back at you and imagine smiling at her.

Mia Scotland
Doula

DID YOU KNOW?

Studies have found that eating six dried dates a day from 32 weeks can help to strengthen the muscles in your uterus to help with delivery.

EXERCISE DURING PREGNANCY

Keeping fit and healthy is vital throughout life, not just when you're pregnant. However, during pregnancy it can be especially beneficial not only for you but also for the health of your baby.

If you have not done much exercise before becoming pregnant, you may want to think about starting. Just make sure that you speak to your doctor or midwife to ensure you've picked a suitable one that you can build up gradually and safely during your pregnancy.

If you already exercise regularly – for example running, swimming or going to a gym – you can, in most cases, continue simply by making a few adjustments.

The benefits of exercise

So why is exercise so good for you when you're pregnant? Firstly, if you're physically fit, you'll have more stamina for when you come to give birth. Many people liken giving birth to doing an endurance event such as a marathon, so if you're fit, you'll be able to keep your energy levels up throughout. Plus, and this may sound strange, exercise can actually make you feel more energetic. If you're fit, the demands of pregnancy, for example carrying the ever-growing bump around, or feeling breathless are less noticeable. Certain exercises can also make you stronger, more supple and flexible, which can be useful during the birth and can speed your recovery afterwards.

Finally, exercise is well known for giving you a natural high thanks to the endorphins – hormones released when you move. These cross the placenta to your baby and make her feel good too.

Swimming

Heading to the pool is a great way to exercise without putting too much strain on yourself.

Swimming can not only help to tone the muscles but the water also gives you a feeling of weightlessness, which can be a great relief when you've been walking around with your large bump all day.

If you opt for swimming, bear in mind that some strokes should be avoided in pregnancy. If you start to suffer from pelvic girdle pain (see page 40), do *not* do breast stroke as the wide movement performed with the legs will aggravate the problem. Once you are into your second trimester, backstroke should be avoided as this could make you feel dizzy (see page 76).

If you're not a fan of swimming lengths, find out if your local pool does any aquanatal classes for pregnancy – basically aerobics classes in the water. They're great because you use the resistance of the water to tone the muscles, but you still have the benefit of feeling weightless in the water. Make sure you choose a class for pregnant women as the instructor will be specially trained in antenatal fitness.

You'll need to buy a proper maternity swimming costume (or a stretchy larger size) to allow for your bump as it grows, or opt for a bikini.

Walking and running

If you've not done much exercise before you became pregnant, walking is perfect as it requires no special skills or abilities. You can just get out there and walk. Best of all, you can fit walking around your everyday life. Try a brisk walk during your lunch break, or get off the bus a stop earlier so you have a bit more of a walk home.

Focus on posture whilst taking your walk, as this will help reduce back pain and relieve any build-up of tension in your neck and shoulders, which can result from sitting at a desk. Wear well-fitting walking shoes or trainers – no loose boots or high heels.

come a time when the bump gets too big, or the weight on your joints becomes uncomfortable. Then you need to start listening to your body and think about swapping running for a low-impact sport such as walking or swimming.

Yoga and Pilates

Both are great for pregnancy, as they focus on building strength and flexibility. It is important you go to a pregnancy-specific class rather a than mainstream one.

Yoga is great for teaching you breathing techniques, which are not only good for relaxation, but they're also useful during labour. Pilates is perfect for staving off back and pelvic pain and for keeping the abdominal muscles strong to help with postnatal recovery.

As for running, this will depend on how much running you did before you got pregnant. You hear about athletes like Paula Radcliffe who continued running for much of their pregnancies. They can do this because it is what they are used to. If you are used to running, say, 20km (12 miles) a week, you could probably continue at least for the first half of your pregnancy. But there will to carry on into late pregnancy, but horses are unpredictable animals that can be spooked by the most innocent of things, so it's probably not worth the risk.

Avoid exercises that involve lying on your back after 16 weeks. The weight of your bump can press on the main blood vessels that carry blood back to the heart, leaving you feeling dizzy and faint.

Be very careful if you undertake high-intensity interval training (HIIT) as it requires you to work at maximal levels of intensity for very short bursts. Current guidelines for pregnancy are to work at moderate levels, although given that one person's moderate is another person's gentle level, the most important thing is to listen to your body.

Sports to avoid

In the first trimester, your uterus is still quite small and protected by the pelvis, so it is possible to continue with most sports. Given that you might not even realize you're pregnant for half of this time, you may not notice a difference in your workout apart from perhaps feeling slightly more tired after exercise than normal.

Once into the second trimester, the top of the uterus will be above the pelvic girdle so it is more exposed and therefore vulnerable. From this point onwards, contact sports or exercise that could see you falling violently or from a height should be avoided. This means stopping ball sports, skiing, horseriding, kick boxing or judo for example. Many passionate horse riders choose

YOUR PELVIC FLOOR

The pelvic floor muscles form a hammock, or sling, of muscles that keep your internal organs pulled in. They are not muscles you are likely to see, but they are muscles you want to exercise, ideally before pregnancy, but definitely during and after pregnancy. They're the muscles responsible for ensuring you remain continent – you can feel them when you need to pee but you're trying to hold it in.

The pelvic floor muscles are extremely important during pregnancy because the urethra (which you pee through), the vagina and the anus all pass through this sling of muscles. Pregnancy and childbirth can weaken the muscles (and that's not to say they're not already weak). The good news is that you can tone and strengthen them through exercise.

The new way to do pelvic floor exercises

In the past, experts would recommend you tone your pelvic floor muscles by simply sitting and squeezing and then releasing them. However, it is now known that the pelvic floor muscles, just like every other muscle in the body, work far better in conjunction with other muscles, such as those in your backside. The latest thinking and advice is that you should incorporate your pelvic floor exercises into other movements, such as lunges, squats and cat stretches and it's been dubbed 'the knack' (see box, right).

EXPERT TIP

GETTING 'THE KNACK' OF YOUR PELVIC FLOOR

The best way to exercise your pelvic floor muscles is to combine it with one the most common movements we do every day – getting up from a seated position and sitting down again.

1. Sit tall with good posture and your feet firmly on the floor between hip and shoulder width apart.

2. Now inhale and then exhale whilst simultaneously fully relaxing your pelvic floor muscles (PFMs).

3. This time, inhale and then as you exhale draw your pelvic floor muscles inwards and upwards while you rise to a standing position. No hands allowed – use your leg muscles to lift yourself up.

4. Now stand tall with good posture and your feet on floor between hip and shoulder width apart.

5. Inhale and then exhale whilst at the same time fully relaxing your pelvic floor muscles.

6. Inhale again, then as you exhale, draw your pelvic floor muscles inwards and upwards as you sit down. Keep your back in a long, neutral position at all times.

Joanna Helcke
Fitness expert

THE SECOND TRIMESTER

MONTH FOUR

Your baby is starting to develop his hearing and eyesight. Soon he will be able to hear your voice and even the sounds of your digestive system.

You'll notice your hair getting thicker and hormones may cause changes in your skin tone too.

WEEK 18

BABY SIZE: BANANA

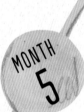

WEEK 19

Your baby's head and facial bones will be formed. Eyes are shut tight and ears can be seen, but don't function yet.

WEEK 16

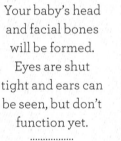

MONTH 5

Your baby's heartbeat can now be heard by your doctor.

WEEK 14

MONTH 4

WEEK 17

His skeleton is mostly rubbery cartilage at this stage, but will start to harden as the weeks go by.

WEEK 15

For many women the earlier side effects such as tiredness and morning sickness will start to subside now, giving you more energy to plan for your growing family.

MONTH FIVE

You'll become more aware of your bump as your baby's weight will double in month five.

You'll have your anomaly scan around this time.

WEEK 20

Your baby's lungs are the least mature organs; they are still filled with amniotic fluid.

WEEK 23

It's important to practise pelvic floor exercises from now on, if you aren't already.

WEEK 25

MONTH 6

WEEK 21

You'll start to feel your baby's first movements.

WEEK 24

WEEK 22

Your breasts may start leaking milk as early as week 22.

WEEK 26

Your bump is getting bigger and you might start to experience backache or leg cramps. You should tell your employer that you're pregnant, if you haven't already.

BABY SIZE: CAULIFLOWER

MONTH SIX

Now's the time to think about which antenatal classes you would like to take. Book one that is close to home as you will be more likely to meet other local mums-to-be.

NOTES

NOTES

YOU ARE WELL OVER HALFWAY THROUGH
YOUR PREGNANCY NOW AND THE FINAL
COUNTDOWN IS READY TO BEGIN.

CHAPTER EIGHT
THIRD TRIMESTER

You're in the home stretch: there's no denying you're pregnant now and your pre-maternity jeans will be firmly pushed to the back of the drawer. You'll be getting seriously excited about the prospect of becoming a mum. Now is the time to start getting yourself organized for when your baby arrives – picking out prams and buggies and marvelling at the tiny babygros, hats and booties that your newborn will be wearing.

MONTH SEVEN

Your baby is growing fast now. In month seven he'll grow from around 36cm (14in) to 40cm (15½in) and he'll start to look more like a newborn. He'll spend most of his time asleep, but he will wake up and move around, stretching and kicking against the walls of your uterus. He may practise other movements such as blinking and sucking his thumb.

ROUTINE TESTS

By this point, you will have had at least two scans and will still be having reasonably regular antenatal appointments. Much like your booking in appointment, these check ups are designed to monitor your health throughout your pregnancy.

- **Blood tests** are carried out at intervals to check your haemoglobin (iron) levels. If there is a risk of anaemia you may be given iron supplements. Your blood sugar levels are checked for signs of gestational diabetes.

- **Urine tests** measure the protein levels in your pee. Presence of proteins could be sign of an infection or of pre-eclampsia.

- **Blood pressure** will be checked at each appointment to monitor for any changes. It is quite normal for your blood pressure to rise slightly during pregnancy. However, a very high reading can be a sign of pre-eclampsia.

How does rhesus status affect a baby?

At your first antenatal appointment, your midwife will have taken a sample of your blood to check your rhesus status. If you and your partner are both rhesus negative there is no risk of problems. However, if you are rhesus negative and your partner is rhesus positive, there's a small chance that your baby will be rhesus positive

too. Having a different blood type to your baby is only an issue if some of your baby's blood enters your bloodstream. This is because your blood cells will treat it as a foreign invader and start producing antibodies against your baby's blood cells. This doesn't matter too much during your first pregnancy, but can affect subsequent pregnancies. If your body produces antibodies against your baby's blood, they remain in your system for life. So if you go on to have another baby that is also rhesus positive, the antibodies can cross the placenta and start attacking your baby's blood cells, which can lead to anaemia in your baby. The good news is that it is easily managed so long as it's picked up at the right time.

Once your midwife has identified that you are rhesus negative, you'll be given injections of a substance known as anti-D. This prevents the body from producing antibodies if you and your baby's blood mixes. The injections are given either as two doses at 28 and 34 weeks, or as one injection at 32 weeks.

When your baby is born, the birthing team will take a sample of blood from the umbilical cord to check his blood type. If it's established that he has a different rhesus status to you, you'll be given a final anti-D injection within 72 hours of the birth. This is because when the placenta separates from your uterus after birth, there's a chance that your baby's blood and your blood could mix. If you have a Caesarean section your blood may also mix with your baby's. If your baby's blood type is the same as yours, you won't need the final anti-D injection.

If your midwife discovers that you already have antibodies in your system at your routine blood test (usually as a result of a previous pregnancy), you won't receive an anti-D injection because it can only prevent antibodies from developing. If they're already there, it won't work. However, a specialist foetal medicine team will monitor your baby to check that he doesn't become anaemic.

It's important that you don't panic too much about the issues surrounding rhesus status, as although it's serious, it's also easily treated as long as you stay up-to-date with check ups.

The glucose tolerance test (GTT)

At one of your first blood tests at the beginning of your pregnancy, your midwife will have checked the levels of sugar in your blood and asked questions to ascertain whether you are at increased risk of gestational (pregnancy) diabetes. Factors such as family history, ethnic origin and being overweight can affect your risk.

If you are at risk, you may be offered a glucose tolerance test (GTT) when you're between 24 and 28 weeks pregnant. This involves having a morning blood test, before you have eaten breakfast, after which you will be given a glucose drink. Two hours later, another blood sample is taken to see how your body deals with the glucose.

If you are diagnosed with gestational diabetes, you may be told to manage the condition with diet (by watching how much sugary food you eat) or with insulin injections. If the condition is not treated properly, you're at an increased risk of premature labour and a larger than average baby.

YOUR BABY'S POSITION

Your baby will move around in your uterus quite a bit before he finally gets too big to do more than just wriggle. With any luck, he'll have settled into a position where his head is down and facing your back and his bottom is pointing towards your head. Babies who lie head up/bottom down are in the breech position which can make delivering them more complicated. There are instances

Q&A

'My baby is in the breech position – could she turn before my due date?'

Midwife **HELEN TAYLOR** says, 'A breech baby means your baby is lying with his head up near your chest and his feet and bottom near the bottom of your womb. It's quite common for a baby to sit like this in the third trimester, but they can also wriggle round to the most common "proper" birth position – head down. Around three in every 100 babies are breech at the end of pregnancy. If your baby is still breech at 36 weeks, you will be offered a scan to check exactly how the baby is lying. Your obstetrician may offer external cephalic version (ECV), in an attempt to manually "turn" your baby round into the right position by manipulating your abdomen. You'll be given special drugs that help to relax the womb muscles first. An ECV works in about half of cases.'

when you can give birth vaginally to a breech baby but it's rare because it carries risks if there isn't a midwife or obstetrician present who is experienced in the correct procedure. If you're adamant that you do want to give birth naturally, talk to your midwife and see if it's possible to have your baby this way.

MATERNITY LEAVE

You should by now have talked to your employer about your maternity leave and what you plan to do. This includes discussing when you'll finish at work and how much time you think you'll take off. Make sure you're aware of your rights when it comes to maternity leave so you can ensure you get treated fairly.

Most pregnant employees are entitled to up to a year's leave – called Statutory Maternity Leave. This is broken down into two halves – the first 26 weeks is called Ordinary Maternity Leave (OML). If you decided to take longer, the next 26 weeks are called Additional Maternity Leave (AML). But you don't have to take the full amount.

Qualifying for maternity leave

Anyone who is pregnant can take Statutory Maternity Leave no matter how long they've been in their job, what they are paid, or the hours they work. But you must tell your employer that you are pregnant no later than the 15th week before the week your baby is due. At the same time, you should advise when your baby is due and when you want to begin your maternity leave.

Maternity leave can commence any time in or after the 11th week before your baby is due. However, your maternity leave will start automatically if you're off work for any reason to do with your pregnancy from the fourth week before your baby is due. Your partner will also be entitled to take leave after the birth of the baby. There are government stipluations and some companies make additonal allowances, so he should check with his HR department.

While you are away from work

Your employer should inform you of anything happening at work that could affect you – this includes opportunities for promotion or job vacancies. But be aware that the amount and type of contact between you and your employer must be reasonable. The way they contact you should also be decided before you leave (for example if you prefer them to reach you by email, phone or have you visit the workplace).

Maternity leave and job security

While you are on leave you will still get all the same rights under your contract of employment as if you were still at work. The only exception is that you will not get your normal pay unless your contract allows for it. But you will, for example, still be entitled to build up holiday and to get any pay increases.

Redundancy

While an employee is on maternity, adoption, paternity or parental leave they have the same redundancy rights as their colleagues; including the right to be offered any suitable alternative

DID YOU KNOW?

You're allowed to work for your employer for up to 10 days during your maternity leave without losing your maternity pay. These are called Keeping in Touch (KIT) days. Not all companies offer KIT days, and they are not obliged to arrange them, nor do you have to take them up. If you take up the offer you'll need to agree a rate of pay with your employer. Some companies stipulate the rate in your contract, others do it on a case-by-case basis, but you must be paid at least the National Minimum Wage.

job if they're selected for redundancy (even if other colleagues are more suitable for the role). An employee can only be made redundant if the employer can clearly justify doing it – for example, a part of the business closes and everyone in that section is made redundant.

Returning to work

Unless you've stated otherwise, your employer will assume you'll be taking your full maternity leave. In which case you don't need to give them notice of when you're coming back (but it might be a good idea to remind them). However, if you decide you want to come back to work before the full year is up, then you'll need to give your employer a period of notice. Check your company's requirments with your HR department. Equally, if you decide not to return to work at all, you must give the normal amount of notice as specified in your employment contract.

MONTH EIGHT

Your bump is well and truly developed (and hopefully you'll be proud to show it off too). Inside, your baby is continuing to grow and develop. The average baby will now be around 48.6cm (19in) long from the top of his head, or crown, to rump, he'll weigh about 2.6kg (5¾lb) and his head is now more in proportion to his body. Your baby's digestive system is now fully functioning, but his intestines are filled with a dark green thick substance called meconium, which is made up of the dead cells and secretions from his bowels. Some babies pass some of this if they become distressed in labour and he will excrete it as his first bowel movements (see page 138–9). His liver, pancreas and kidneys are all working, and any urine your baby produces will be excreted into your amniotic fluid.

Nesting

It's normal at this stage and in the last few weeks before your due date to have the sudden urge to clean out all your kitchen cupboards, wash and fold every single item of baby clothing and paint the bathroom. Welcome to nesting – a common reaction for many pregnant women as they prepare to meet their baby.

Nesting is a primal reaction to the impending birth. You may normally *hate* cleaning or tidying, but being pregnant turns you into a mother hen who wants to feather her nest and make it perfect for her baby chick's arrival.

If you do decide the house needs to be cleaned from top to bottom, bear in mind that some cleaning products aren't suitable during pregnancy, particularly if there's a risk of you inhaling them (so, for example, leave cleaning the oven to your other half).

If you want to bypass chemical cleaning products now you're pregnant, try using natural items you'll find around the house, such as lemon juice, bicarbonate of soda, vinegar and salt. For example, mixing up a paste of lemon juice, bicarbonate of soda and salt makes a great scouring cream to make taps and draining boards shine. Vinegar and water make a great window cleaning solution.

DRESSING YOUR BUMP

By now you'll probably have a sizeable bump and you may have your clothes sorted. But if you're struggling to know how to dress your bump so you don't feel like you're swimming in circus tent tops, or spend a fortune on clothes you won't be wearing for very long there are some tips you can follow.

Keep your personal style

If you're a fan of pencil skirts and fitted jumpers pre-pregnancy, there's nothing to say you can't keep this trend going now. Many high street shops have a great range of clothes with stretchy fit material or panels to accommodate your growing bump. Remember that fitted clothes will show off your bump and emphasize it. If you try to swamp it in enormous clothes, you'll look even bigger than you are.

Bump up your dress size

If you love a top or dress but it's not available in the shop's maternity range, see if you can get away with buying a couple of sizes up. Go for shift dresses and shirts, as you can belt them up post-baby to pull the waist in.

Invest in one key maternity item

Whether it's a fantastic maternity coat or a great pair of maternity jeans, if you spend a bit of money on one item, you can then dress all your other clothes around it.

QUICK FIX

· · · · · · · · · · · · · · ·

SHOW OFF YOUR CURVES

If pregnancy has seen you grow in the bust department, don't be afraid to embrace it with lower necklines (although watch out if your work has a strict dress policy) – a v-neck or sweetheart neckline works best. Plus, it will help distract from your swollen ankles!

Discover your accessories

Statement necklaces, scarves, belts and hair pieces are ideal when you're pregnant as you'll be able to jazz up a plain item with them throughout your pregnancy and beyond. They'll also help you maintain your pre-baby identity no matter what your size or shape.

SEX WITH A BUMP

As we already explained in chapter six, your libido could be subject to ups and downs during pregnancy. Some women get a boost, while others lose interest completely. This also applies to your partner. Some people worry that it is not safe to have sex in pregnancy; the good news is that it is perfectly safe and it can be positively beneficial. It helps you maintain (and even build on) your relationship with your partner and it can help you both unwind.

If you decide to use sex toys during pregnancy, make sure they're thoroughly cleaned before you use them otherwise you risk admitting bacteria into your vagina, which could be potentially harmful. Most importantly, make sure you let your partner know if something is uncomfortable. It might take some trial and error to find a position that works for you both. As pregnancy can cause problems and pain with hips, knees or back, you and your partner may want to explore what is comfortable for you. Most positions are possible in the early months, but as your bump grows you may not want your partner to rest on it – he may not want to either. Your breasts may be very tender too.

It is okay to have sex for short periods if that's all you feel comfortable with, or for sex not to end in orgasm every time. It is also okay to not have sex at all if you are too uncomfortable to really enjoy it. The good news is that pregnancy also allows you to explore your body in other ways and experience new feelings of pleasure and different ways to enjoy sex you might not have tried before.

QUICK FIX

COMFORTABLE SEX

Make use of pillows, chairs, the bed or a table if you need extra support during sex and don't feel like you have to stay in the same position throughout, as it may start to get uncomfortable.

Q&A

'My partner has lost interest in having sex with me now i'm pregnant. should i be worried?'

Sex and relationships expert **DR PETRA BOYNTON** says, 'Not at all. Women often assume that men want sex all the time, but during pregnancy, the relationship dynamic can change, which when you're feeling particularly vulnerable, can be difficult. It can be tempting to assume that the reason he doesn't want to have sex is your fault, but your partner is going through some very big emotional changes of his own as he gets used to the idea of being a father. He may worry that he'll hurt you, or the baby, or find it strange to feel the baby moving during sex. If this is the case, there are still ways for you to feel close as a couple. You could try massage, oral sex or kissing and cuddles. Sit down and talk about your concerns, that way you can work out whether there's anything else you can do, or whether you just want to not worry about it.'

MONTH NINE

It's been a long time coming, and you will probably be feeling so excited yet nervous about meeting your baby that you could burst. Your bump will probably be so big it looks like you are ready to pop. You may be feeling quite uncomfortable now, because your baby has become very big and it's more difficult for you to move around. This is when becoming a mum suddenly starts feeling real. You may also notice the muscles of your uterus tightening a few times a day – these are Braxton Hicks contractions (it's not labour) and can be felt any time from 16 weeks.

Your baby's head may have moved down into your pelvis now, making it more uncomfortable for you; when this happens it is said to be 'engaged'. You may notice that your bump moves down a little. Sometimes, however, the baby's head doesn't engage until labour starts. If you haven't packed your hospital bag yet, it's worth doing so now, just in case you get caught unawares. Turn to page 105 for ideas on what to pack.

Be aware of your baby's movements

You may notice that your baby is not moving around as much. Make sure you keep an eye on his movements. While previously, it was recommended that you 'count the kicks', all babies are different and don't all move about in the same way or the same amount. Some mums may be so busy doing things that they do not notice when their baby is kicking, and then worry when they feel no movement. A better plan is to just stay aware of your baby's normal movement patterns. Your baby may move a lot at night, or when you're in the bath – so look out for his 'kicks' then. If you haven't felt your baby move for a couple of hours, stop what you're doing and lie down for 20 minutes. A gentle prod of your stomach or drinking a glass of cold water may also wake him up. If you're at all worried talk to your midwife.

Pregnancy dreams

Been having some frankly downright bizarre dreams recently? Don't worry, you're not the first. Experiencing strange dreams in pregnancy is extremely common. Nobody's quite sure what causes them, but it could be related to your hormones. Alternatively it could be because you have a lot on your mind and the dreams are your brain's way of processing your thoughts. Talk to your partner if you're anxious about your dreams.

GOING OVERDUE

Your due date may be etched into your brain but there is no guarantee that your baby will arrive then. The date is worked out from the first day of your last period but, in reality, this is more of a guideline and your baby could easily be born

EXPERT TIP

....

GET A HEAD START FOR LABOUR

Sit on an exercise ball for two lots of 20 minutes a day. It's great for encouraging 'optimal foetal positioning' for labour.

Helen Taylor
Midwife

before or after what's predicted. In fact, labour begins naturally any time between 37 and 42 weeks in most pregnancies.

If things haven't started and you're past your due date, there are a variety of activities and actions that might kickstart labour. Go for a long walk, as walking can help to move your baby into the right position for birth. The head may engage, which can get things moving. Acupuncture and reflexology use needles or pressure to stimulate the body's energy to get your uterus to contract. Make sure you visit a registered practitioner who is qualified to work with pregnant women.

Try eating pineapple or go for a curry. There's not actually any proof that these foods can help to start labour, but there's no harm in trying. Pineapple contains bromelain, which is said to help soften your cervix. A spicy curry will stimulate your tummy, and some women swear it has a knock-on effect on their uterus, too. Just bear in mind that very spicy curry could also give you heartburn, so if you've been suffering from this, it might be worth giving it a miss.

Can sex trigger labour?

There is some debate as to whether sex can actually trigger labour. While it was previously believed that your partner's sperm contains prostaglandins that can help to soften the cervix and start labour, a Malaysian study in 2012 found there was no connection between the two. Of course, that's not to say you can't try having sex if you want to. The contractions you'll get during an orgasm may very well do the job of starting labour. In addition nipple stimulation is thought to trigger the release of oxytocin, the hormone that causes contractions to start – a great activity for your partner to get involved in.

EXPERT TIP

SEX IN LATER STAGES

It sounds strange, but many of the sex positions that you can try during pregnancy are similar to those you can take in childbirth. So if you're thinking about birthing positions, you could bring these into your sex life. Mix it up to prevent unnecessary aches. This applies whether you are having penetrative sex or enjoying other pleasures like oral sex or masturbation.

If your partner is used to intimacy leading to sex, it can be difficult to explain that, yes, you really do just want a hug. If you're concerned kisses will develop into something more that you're uncomfortable with, set ground rules with your partner beforehand. Explain that, when you want sex, you'll tell him, or if you feel too shy to initiate sex that you'll both agree if he asks but if you say no he'll respect that. It means you can maintain intimacy without having to push him away. Alternatively it may be you who wants sex a lot more and will need to accept that what he'd prefer is a hug. Being affectionate is a good habit to get into now. When the baby arrives, little gestures will get you through the first few months when it's much harder to find time for yourselves.

Dr Petra Boynton
Sex and relationships expert

BEING INDUCED

If you go overdue (usually after a week), your midwife may offer you a sweep. He or she will run her finger around your cervix to attempt to separate the membranes of the amniotic sac from the cervix. This will release a hormone that helps bring on labour. A sweep can be uncomfortable, so you may need to take some paracetamol to ease any cramps you may experience. If nothing has happened you'll probably be offered a second sweep 48 hours later. If you still haven't gone into labour, your midwife may suggest an induction. Likewise, if your waters have broken naturally, but your contractions haven't started, you may need to be induced. This is because there is an increased risk of infection now that the amniotic sac is no longer acting as a protective cover for your baby.

The first stage of induction is to insert a pessary containing prostaglandins to help prepare the cervix for birth. Your midwife or doctor may also break your waters using a small hook that looks a bit like a knitting needle; this is usually done after the pessary (and only if your cervix is wide enough to allow it). If this doesn't work, you may be put on a syntocinon drip. Syntocinon is the artificial version of oxytocin, the hormone your body releases to stimulate contractions. Once labour begins, you'll be offered pain relief (see page 114) as the pain can come on quite strongly.

REAL LIFE

'Acupuncture triggered my labour'

'When my due date came and went, I wasn't too worried. It was my first baby and people kept telling me that they are usually late. I tried all the usual things to bring on labour – curry, long walks – but nothing happened. My midwife gave me a sweep and still nothing. She said I could come in for another one in a day or so, but they'd need to start thinking about induction as I was over a week late. I was desperate to not be induced, so looked into acupuncture. The acupuncturist inserted very fine needles at different points in the body; it didn't hurt and was actually very relaxing. She showed me some acupressure points that I could massage myself. I had a second session two days later – the day before I was due to have an induction. This time I could feel my womb contracting and four hours later I was in full labour. A total success!'

LINDSAY, MUM TO TOMMY, 14 MONTHS

DID YOU KNOW?

You can refuse an induction, but remember that while your baby is still growing beyond 40 weeks, your placenta is not, and this could affect the nutrient and blood supply to your baby. You can ask for a scan to check the health and wellbeing of your baby and placenta. Once you go 14 days overdue, most hospitals urge you to have an induction.

THE THIRD TRIMESTER

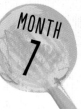

MONTH 7

Stretch marks may start to appear on your tummy and breasts.

WEEK 28

WEEK 27

Your baby can now open his eyes.

Your belly button might start to protrude, but it will return to normal after the birth.

WEEK 30

WEEK 29

Your baby is becoming more sensitive to light, taste, sound and smell. He can sense light through the wall of your uterus.

MONTH 8

WEEK 32

WEEK 31

Your baby is about to start his final growth spurt.

Your baby is growing rapid[ly] and he's gettin[g] rounder as he starts to lay fat stores underneath h[is] skin.

WEEK 34

WEEK 33

BABY SIZE: HONEYDEW MELON

MONTH SEVEN

Your baby will be about 40cm (14½in) long by the end of this month and will be wriggling and kicking in your belly so you'll really be aware he's there.

MONTH EIGHT

You may suddenly find yourself with an urge to clean your home from top to bottom, wash all the baby clothes and make sure everything's ready and in place for his arrival.

MONTH NINE

You'll find that you're getting to recognize your baby's movements now; what wakes him up and gets him moving, although his movements will start to lessen as the space in your uterus becomes more cramped as your baby gets bigger. Try to stay aware of your baby's normal movement pattern and talk to your midwife straight away if you're at all worried.

WEEK 35

MONTH 9

WEEK 36

If your baby is born at 37 weeks, he will not be considered premature but his immune system is still developing.

WEEK 37

Make sure your hospital bag is packed by now if you haven't packed it already.

WEEK 38

You might start to experience Braxton Hicks contractions.

WEEK 39

WEEK 40

Your due date is calculated at 40 weeks but in reality fewer than five per cent of babies are born on their due date.

WEEK 41

WEEK 42

If your baby hasn't been born, options for being induced will be discussed.

NOTES

NOTES

YOU ARE NEARLY THERE. GET READY FOR
THE MOST EXCITING BIT — MEETING YOUR
BABY AT LAST!

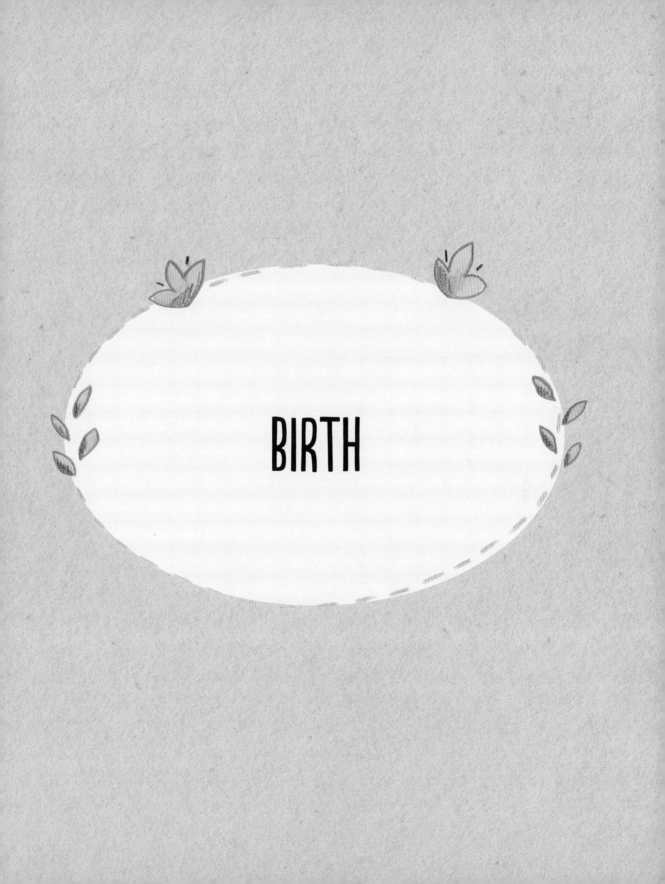

BIRTH

CHOOSING WHAT KIND OF HOSPITAL AND
MEDICAL SUPPORT YOU NEED DURING THE BIRTH

CREATING YOUR BIRTH PLAN

PICKING AND PREPARING YOUR BIRTH PARTNER

PACKING YOUR HOSPITAL BAG AND ENSURING
YOU HAVE EVERYTHING THAT YOU, YOUR
PARTNER AND YOUR BABY WILL NEED
ON THE BIG DAY

CHAPTER NINE
PREPARING FOR BIRTH

There's a reason pregnancy is nine months long,
and it isn't just for growing your baby. As well as
picking out the perfect cot or buggy and coming
to terms with how you're actually going to get this
baby out (without dwelling on that *too* much),
you've got to prepare yourself and your partner
mentally and physically for the actual birth.
Once you've decided on where you want to give
birth, think about writing your birth plan and
decide on who is going to be your birth partner.

PICKING YOUR BIRTH LOCATION

Deciding where you'll deliver your baby is one of the biggest decisions you'll make as it can influence who delivers your baby and the type of pain relief available. But how do you know what is right for you?

The good news is that you have more choices than you think – with the basic options of home, a midwife-led unit or hospital. It's a good idea to do your research and visit the hospital (or hospitals if there are more nearby) and midwife unit to weigh up your options. Consider journey time to get there (in traffic) and go for the place that you feel can help you have the birth that best suits you and your pregnancy.

Hospital birth

A hospital maternity ward has the most clinical atmosphere, but that doesn't have to mean bright lights and whirring machines. Even on the main labour ward, the equipment is sometimes tucked away in 'bedroom' furniture and you can switch off some of the lights. You will have a midwife looking after you, but you'll also have access to other health professionals such as doctors and anaesthetists, and importantly the greatest variety of pain relief. Many NHS hospitals do have at least one birthing pool, but there is no guarantee it will be available when you start labour.

Hospital is a good option if you want to try all forms of pain relief and/or you are anxious about the birth and prefer to have doctors nearby. If you have a high-risk pregnancy (see right) you'll be advised to go for a hospital birth. However, NHS hospitals are also extremely busy and if

EXPERT TIP

ARE YOU HAVING A HIGH-RISK PREGNANCY?

Your pregnancy is considered a high risk if:

- You're carrying two or more babies.

- You're aged over 40 or a teenager.

- Your baby is in the breech or transverse (side-to-side) position.

- You have a medical condition such as diabetes, gestational diabetes or a clotting disorder.

- You have Group B strep – a type of bacteria present in some women that can cause infection in newborns.

- You have high blood pressure.

- You're overweight.

- You've previously had a Caesarean delivery.

- You lost a lot of blood in a previous delivery.

- You have cysts on your ovaries or fibroids in your womb.

- You have a history of repeated miscarriages.

- Previous babies were small-for-dates, or very big.

- You've delivered a previous baby early.

- You've conceived through IVF.

Shreelata Datta
Obstetrician

you have a long labour you are likely to have different midwives during your labour because of shift changes. If you want continuous one-to-one support, especially during the first stage of labour, you may want to opt for a home birth.

You can opt for a private hospital, but it is expensive. Plus you will have to pay extra for medication, and this includes an epidural. However, you will see the same consultant throughout your pregnancy, you'll have control over how you give birth, one-on-one care during labour, and hotel-like surroundings and access to a breastfeeding consultant post-birth.

There's some debate about whether the birth is more medicalized in private hospitals because the obstetricians are so ready to hand, but it does depend on how your birth is going. If you don't want or need an obstetrician during your birth, then he doesn't have to be there; you will have a midwife throughout. Some private hospitals have midwife-led units attached to them where a team of midwives will look after you with obstetricians available in the background if there's a problem.

Midwife-led unit

These aim to recreate a home-from-home experience, often with birth pools and spacious delivery rooms. The units are staffed by midwives, and some are attached to a hospital. If you have a slow labour or complications you will be transferred to a hospital delivery suite. If the unit is attached to a hospital the transfer will be relatively quick and easy, if it's a stand-alone unit, you'll be taken by ambulance.

The emphasis at midwife-led units is on natural birth and you are limited to gas and air and pethidine for pain relief. If you find you want an epidural, you'll need to be to moved to the hospital. A midwife-led unit is ideal if you want a more relaxed atmosphere, but are not

comfortable with a home birth. However, if you're considered 'high-risk' (see page 99) you may not be able to deliver in a midwife-led unit.

Home birth

Picking this option means you'll have your baby where you are most comfortable. You can hire a birthing pool, light candles and walk from room to room and a community midwife will be on hand to deliver your baby. Pain relief options are the same as in a midwife-led unit and you will be transferred to hospital by ambulance if things don't go to plan. Around a third of women who choose a home birth go to hospital, but it's often for an epidural or failure to progress.

A home birth is fine for straightforward pregnancies and also for second and subsequent births, and ideal if you crave home comforts and want a familiar midwife. But if you would prefer the security of immediate access to doctors, medical equipment and an epidural, you may prefer a hospital. It's worth noting that 2014 guidance from the National Institute for Health and Care Excellence (NICE) recommends that giving birth in midwife-led units or at home is *safer* than hospital births for low-risk mums-to-be who are having second or subsequent babies, because there's less risk of medical intervention.

WRITING A BIRTH PLAN

Although it's not compulsory, it can be a good idea to write down what you'd like to happen during your birth. This is so your midwife knows how you'd like your labour to progress and she can support you in your choices.

Make sure that you are prepared for all eventualities and that you understand the different medical interventions available to you. Sometimes childbirth takes an unexpected turn and it's best to make sure that your midwife and birth partner are clear what your ideal birth is as well as what your preferences are if there needs to be a change of plan.

When to start
You'll probably want to start thinking about your birth plan when you are around 32 weeks pregnant. This gives you the chance to consider your options and ask plenty of questions about labour and birth in advance from your midwife or antenatal teacher or teachers.

Imagine your perfect birth setting
Try to visualize yourself giving birth to help you decide how you want it to go. We're not talking about you sneezing your baby out while your hair stays perfectly in place in less than hour (you've got to be a little bit realistic). This is more so you can link your feelings and experiences. Imagine you're in labour feeling full of confidence and what things will help you feel that way – the people around you, the environment you're in. Put this in your plan.

Consider pain relief
Whether you want to give birth as naturally as possible, or you think you'd prefer every kind of pain relief available, it pays to stay open-minded. In your birth plan, rate your preferences in order

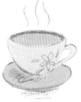

REAL LIFE

'I was making tea during labour'

'I decided to give birth to my second child at home. I felt very relaxed as I was making myself cups of tea and pottering about during labour. I also got to sleep in my own bed on the first night with my son and husband close by.'

**GAIL, MUM TO EMMA,
FOUR AND TOM, TWO**

– for example, say you'll start with TENS machine and you would like a birthing pool with gas and air if necessary. You would like pethidine only if it gets very uncomfortable. You would opt for an epidural only if things get more painful than you'd like.

Remember that pain-relief options depend on where you give birth. There's no point asking for a birthing pool if your chosen hospital doesn't have one. Similarly, if you've elected to give birth at a midwife-led unit, an epidural won't be an option, because it needs to be administered by a hospital anaesthetist. Chat to your midwife about your options, as he or she will know what's on offer.

How would you feel about a Caesarean section

This may not be top of your wish list, but it's wise to know what it involves as 25 per cent of babies are born this way. Think about what you would like to happen in case a Caesarean becomes necessary on the day. For example, would you prefer a spinal block or epidural rather than a general anaesthetic and would you still like to delay cutting the cord (page 125).

Pick your birth music

If you feel soothed by music, listening to your favourite album may help you relax. Make sure you pack battery-operated speakers or have a phone that plays music well as you may not be able to plug in a music player or iPod dock in your birthing room. On the other hand, find out if your labour room already has somewhere to plug in music as that's one less thing to pack in your hospital bag.

After you've given birth

Most hospitals give you an injection to speed up the third stage of labour, which is when your placenta is delivered. If you'd prefer to deliver it naturally, make this clear. A birth plan is also not just for labour – it's also a good way to outline how you'd like to spend those precious first few minutes after your baby has been born. Do you want to see the sex for yourself or be told? Do you want to wait a few minutes before the cord is clamped? Does your partner want to cut the cord? Do you want your baby to be cleaned up or placed straight on you for skin-to-skin contact? Write it all down.

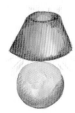

REAL LIFE

'The midwife-led birth centre provided everything we needed'

'I felt so lucky planning the birth as my nearest hospital had a great midwife-led birth centre tacked onto the side of it. My sister had her baby there, so I knew it was going to be right for us. As my due date approached, we had a tour of the facilities they had available, which included comfy rooms with pools for water births, birth balls and mats, plus somewhere for my partner to stay comfortable during the birth. When I went into labour and headed to the centre I was able to slip into a warming birthing pool, where I stayed for several hours. The midwives were totally supportive and friendly the whole time. After a while, I decided to get out and just lean over a birth ball while kneeling on a mat. The atmosphere was so relaxing, with dimmed lights and no beeping machines, that I felt great, even during the tough pushing stage. Afterwards, my partner and I snuggled up on the bed with Isla.'

JOANNA, MUM TO ISLA, FOUR MONTHS

PREPARING YOUR BIRTH PARTNER

Chances are, the person you'll want with you during labour will be your partner. You may be allowed two birth partners, but check with your chosen hospital or unit what their policy is. If you end up having a Caesarean, you will only be allowed one birth partner in the operating room. Having decided on a birth partner you need to help him or her to prepare for your baby's birth.

Does the father want to be there?
Today's modern man almost always takes an active role during birth. In fact, only 5 per cent of fathers are not present in the delivery room, which is a massive change from the births of thirty years ago. But if your partner isn't comfortable – many men admit they struggle to see their partner in so much pain – then it's best not to force him as it could end up leaving you feeling more stressed. Just make sure you discuss this *before* he passes out in the delivery room, and be flexible. You may think you don't want a particular person as your birth partner, and then change your mind as the day nears.

How can my birth partner help during labour?
You'll probably both get a good idea about this after going to antenatal classes, but it will also depend on how involved you want your partner to be and how much he or she feels comfortable doing. You can teach them massage techniques to help ease your back pain, or show them how to help you hold birth positions. You may want them to get in the birth pool too. Then again, you might prefer that they simply stay next to you, hold your hand and provide words of support or some light relief (although be warned, those funny jokes that your partner likes to tell may not be quite so funny in the middle of a contraction).

Q&A

'I'm not sure if I want my husband to be with me during labour. How do I tell him?'

Doula **MIA SCOTLAND** says, 'If you don't want your partner to be with you during labour, it's important you take this seriously. Don't have him with you just because you feel you should. Your feelings during birth matter, because if you feel uncomfortable, self-conscious or stressed, it will not help your labour. When you talk to him, don't focus on what he might do wrong (for example, "you'll make me tense"). Focus on what is good in your relationship, and that you want to keep it that way ("I love that you find me sexy, and I want to keep it that way" or "your help is really important, and I want you strong and refreshed when our baby is born so you can really support me after"). If you both agree that he is not going to be there, you still need to decide on his role – when he will see you and the baby, whether he will be in the corridor or at home, how he can be helpful in the time before you go to the hospital.'

Does your birth partner know and understand your plan?

A good birth partner is one that can act as your advocate during labour, especially if you are not able to respond. That means knowing when you need him or her to fight your corner. They need to understand the different types of pain relief and when you want them to come into play. At the same time, they need to be able to pick up on when you've changed your mind. Decide too if your partner will take a specific role during labour, such as cutting the cord or even catching the baby (yes really!). Some partners enjoy being very hands on while others may not feel comfortable and prefer to take more of a back seat.

Do you want a second birth partner?

This may be a good idea as it means the two of them can 'tag team' and give each other breaks. The last thing you want is to be going through a particularly strong contraction while in need of your partner's support when he's nipped out to use the toilet or get a coffee. If your labour is particularly long, one birth partner can provide support while the other can get a sandwich or put more money in the parking meter.

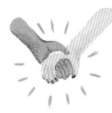

REAL LIFE

'My boyfriend stayed near my head'

'My partner was a complete rock during birth. He got me snacks, massaged my back, fanned me when I was hot and barely left my side. But there was one thing he was adamant on — he didn't want to be near the "business end" during labour. He's very squeamish and was worried he'd pass out if he saw anything. I was fine with this as he'd warned me before.'

NICOLA, MUM TO OLLY, SIX MONTHS

EXPERT TIP

TOP 3 HOSPITAL BAG ITEMS

1. Nutritious snacks for labour — think slow release carbohydrates such as oatcakes and dried fruit or bananas for energy.

2. It might not fit in your hospital bag, but it might be worth taking in one of your own pillows for support in labour as they can be in short supply in hospital and it's good to have something familiar to lean up against.

3. Sports-top water bottles — they're much easier to drink out of when in labour than trying to sip from a cup and it's very important to stay well-hydrated in labour.

Helen Taylor
Midwife

PACKING YOUR HOSPITAL BAGS

If you've got your newborn's kit sorted, it's time to start thinking about what you want to take with you if you're giving birth in a hospital or birth centre (and even if you're having a home birth, being prepared for a trip to hospital). It's best to start getting things together about a month before your due date and have a bag packed at least three weeks before. But what do you need to pack to keep you going and your partner happy?

CHECK OFF THESE ITEMS SO YOU'VE GOT ALL BASES COVERED:

FOR YOUR BABY

☐ Baby clothes such as vests, sleepsuits, scratch mitts and a hat and an all-in-one for going home.

☐ Newborn nappies – some hospitals provide them, but bring spare just in case – and cotton wool.

☐ Bottles and formula if you're going to bottle feed.

FOR YOUR BIRTH PARTNER

☐ Camera (with disc space) and a charger.

☐ Snacks for him.

☐ Change of clothes, so if your labour is very long he won't need to go home to change. Take swimming shorts in case he gets into the pool.

☐ iPad or book so that if you have a snooze (thanks epidural), your partner has something to do.

☐ Travel pillow in case you're both trying to get some sleep and he's only got a chair.

FOR YOU

☐ TENS machine can help relieve early labour pain (see page 111).

☐ Portable speaker (with batteries) to play your labour playlist.

☐ A T-shirt or comfortable top to wear in labour if you want to.

☐ Warm bed socks as it's not unusual for your feet to feel a bit cold in labour as all the blood is headed towards your uterus to help it dilate.

☐ Hair ties to keep hair out of your face.

☐ Lip balm as using gas and air can sometimes make lips quite dry.

☐ Wash bag with toothbrush and toothpaste – pack gentle perfume- and colour-free shower gel for your first post-baby shower.

☐ Nursing bra and pads as your breasts can be quite uncomfortable as the milk begins to come in.

☐ Comfortable knickers – now is not the time for your favourite lacy thong.

☐ Ultra-absorbent sanitary towels – you'll be bleeding quite heavily for at least the first few days, if not longer.

☐ Comfy post-labour clothes – think tracksuit bottoms, hoodie and trainers (only Victoria Beckham walks out in designer shoes).

CHAPTER TEN
THE SIGNS OF LABOUR

Your bag is packed, you've cooked and frozen enough food to last a month, vacuumed every corner of the house and can't remember the last time you could see your toes. You're now anxiously looking out for those first pangs of labour. While your body has been gearing up for birth from the moment you become pregnant, it's now that you'll notice things shifting into gear. Many women expect there to be a sudden rush of signs like you see on the TV, but it's often a slow build-up.

THE EARLY SIGNS YOUR BABY IS NEARLY HERE

The first indications that your baby is about to arrive aren't really labour signs as such, but more an indication that everything is progressing as it should be in the last couple of weeks. They might not seem particularly noticeable or special, and don't worry about them. Simply embrace them as the final part of your amazing pregnancy journey.

Leaky nipples

Your breasts start producing milk even before you give birth, so you may discover wet patches on your bra in the days leading up to your due date. The liquid is colostrum, a nutrient-rich 'milk' that will nourish your baby until your proper milk comes in a couple of days after birth. Nipples can leak throughout the final trimester, but you'll probably notice it most in the last few weeks before your baby arrives. Wear breast pads in your bra to soak up milk if necessary.

The pregnancy waddle

If your gait has started to resemble a cross between a cowboy and a duck – half shuffle, half sway, then it's probably a sign that your baby will soon be arriving. Your pelvis widens in preparation for birth, which can affect the way you walk. Your legs will seem further apart and this coupled with a big bump, can mean you walk with a side-to-side rocking movement. If the change in gait is accompanied with pain, it could be pelvic girdle pain (see PGP, page 42).

Swollen down below

Pregnancy has a tendency to leave you feeling swollen in different places, including your labia and the entrance to your vagina. It can be a bit disconcerting, but it's very normal. When your baby moves down into your pelvis, generally after week 37, it also puts more pressure on the veins around your vagina, making the area feel swollen. Ease any discomfort by placing an ice pack in a clean tea towel and resting it on the area.

A burst of energy

If getting up off the sofa is about as much activity as you can manage for most of your last trimester, the sudden burst of energy that you get in the days before labour starts (and the urge to clean out your kitchen cupboards) could take you by surprise. Nobody's really sure why women get this boost, but it could be their body gearing up for labour. If you can't sit still, use this time to finish off odd jobs, do some cooking or see friends. Equally, if the energy burst doesn't arrive, don't worry. It's better to conserve your energy for the most important bit – giving birth.

EXPERT TIP

PACK CHRONOLOGICALLY

The last thing you want is to have to empty your hospital bag trying to find hair ties or your water bottle, so put what you'll need first near the top; put your going home clothes and sanitary towels at the bottom. Pack clothes for your newborn in a separate compartment. Make sure your birth partner knows where everything is, so he does not have tip the bag up to find what you need.

Mia Scotland
Doula

EXPERT TIP

BRAXTON HICKS V. LABOUR PAINS – HOW CAN YOU TELL THE DIFFERENCE?

Braxton Hicks are like practice contractions. They're designed to tone up your uterus ready for the real deal. You can tell the difference between Braxton Hicks and real contractions because the former aren't usually painful. You'll notice your stomach hardening, but labour contractions become increasingly stronger, more frequent and more painful, while Braxton Hicks won't.

Helen Taylor
Midwife

ARE YOU IN LABOUR?

There's no set pattern to labour and you may notice all of the following signs, or you may only have a couple, but once you spot them, you'll know that things are starting. Just remember, labour starts gently and gradually develops over hours – even days – before your baby arrives.

Backache

An ache in your lower back can mean your baby is lying with her back to yours and rotating into the right position for labour. This can take a few days and may be painful. Or it could be the start of your contractions – some women experience them more in their back than their stomach.

You can ease the discomfort by taking the recommended dose of paracetamol, taking a warm bath, or asking your partner for a back rub.

Your waters break

This happens when the sac of amniotic fluid surrounding the baby ruptures. You may feel a huge gush, or have a slow trickle that lasts a few days. Remember, your waters can break at any time during labour or birth and may even remain intact well into established labour.

When this happens, grab a sanitary towel then call the maternity unit. A midwife will ask you about the fluid: it should be a straw-like colour and have a sweet odour. If it's green, your baby has emptied her bowels and you'll need to go straight to hospital to check for infection. Otherwise, stay at home – your labour is likely to start within the next 72 hours. If your waters break but you haven't felt any contractions in those first 24 hours, talk to your midwife as you may need to be induced (see page 91).

You have a 'show' in your knickers

This is the mucus plug that sits inside the neck of the cervix during pregnancy to prevent bacteria getting into the womb. As your cervix starts to dilate, the plug will come out and will look blood-tinged and jelly-like. It may come out either in one go or in bits. If this happens, speak to your midwife to check it's a show and you're not just bleeding. Then eat, sleep and relax.

You feel contractions

Real contractions start off quite weak, almost like period pains, and will grow in intensity. You may feel your stomach harden and the feeling will come in a wave that builds in intensity. However, women feel contractions differently. Many tell you that labour is *nothing* like period pains, while others will claim that early labour bears some similarity to bad period pains.

EXPERT TIP

HOW TO TIME A CONTRACTION

Using a stopwatch (or an app on your phone), press start as soon as your tummy muscles begin to harden. Click stop once the contraction has faded, and you'll have the length. Hit start again straightaway then wait until you feel another contraction begin — now you know how far apart they are. Keep timing like this for about 30 minutes so you know how long your contractions are and whether they're increasing in frequency. This is a good job for your birth partner to do.

Helen Taylor
Midwife

Q&A

'I've had pregnancy heartburn for months, but it's eased off. Why?'

Midwife **HELEN TAYLOR** says, 'This is because your baby has dropped, which means he's moved down into your pelvis ready for birth. This can happen any time from 37 weeks, right up until just before you go into labour. You may find you can breathe more easily, as your baby isn't pushing against your lungs and decreasing their capacity. You could also notice a heavy sensation lower down in your pelvis.'

Real contractions will grow in frequency (unlike Braxton Hicks). When you feel contractions, don't rush to hospital as you may be sent home, but do let the unit know what's happening. Try to relax, distract yourself with a DVD or odd jobs or take a bath. You can take a paracetamol or use your TENS machine (see page 111) to cope with early labour pain. Labour is usually considered established when you have three one-minute contractions within ten minutes. When the contractions become so intense you struggle to talk, you'll know it's definitely time to head to hospital.

CHAPTER ELEVEN
PAIN RELIEF

When it comes to labour, whether you decide to
wait as long as possible before asking for pain relief,
or demand your epidural as soon as you arrive at
hospital, it's very important you find out what's
available to you.

WHAT ARE THE OPTIONS?

There are a number of different options available to you and it's very much your choice. Many women think they would like to go without pain relief in labour, but it's very common to have some kind of help. A few women manage with no assistance and some have everything going. Labour is not an endurance test and pain relief is there to help you if you need it.

Paracetamol

When you start feeling the first pangs of labour, you can take the recommended dose of paracetamol to ease the pain and aches. Depending on your pain threshold, this may not make any difference, but for some it's enough to keep going until they need to go into hospital.

TENS machine

Another useful early labour pain relief tool is a TENS, 'transcutaneous electrical nerve stimulation', machine. You attach four sticky pads to your back and wires send out electrical pulses that block pain messages as they travel through nerves to your brain. The pulses encourage your body to release feel-good endorphins, thought to be natural pain relievers. Hospitals don't tend to have TENS machines, but you can easily buy your own or hire one for up to four weeks. Ask around and see if any friends have one you could borrow.

Some women find TENS machines very effective, while others don't experience any results – you really just have to try it and see how you go. The good news is that you're in charge and can regulate the degree of stimulation and it has no known side effects to either you or your baby, but remember they're battery operated so you won't be able to use them if you want to get into a bath or birthing pool.

EXPERT TIP

USING GAS AND AIR EFFECTIVELY

Do ask the midwife looking after you in labour to give you directions on how to use gas and air, but essentially, as soon as you know you have another contraction coming, start using the gas as there's a 10 to 15 second delay before it starts working. By the time the contraction has built up in strength, you should be feeling the benefits.

Helen Taylor
Midwife

Gas and air

Entonox, which is commonly known as gas and air, is available in all birth centres and hospitals and can also be administered to you at home by your midwife if you opt for a home birth.

Also known as 'laughing gas', gas and air is made up of 50 percent oxygen and 50 percent nitrous oxide, and it helps to take the edge off the pain, rather than blocking it out altogether. Some women find it makes them relaxed or happy, while others find they can feel light-headed and nauseous. The benefit of gas and air is that you have total control and it's easy to start and stop when you want. You simply hold a mouthpiece attached to the main supply and breathe in deeply when a contraction begins. And while the effects

DON'T FORGET

Pack lip balm and water as using gas and air can leave you with a dry mouth and lips, which can be uncomfortable.

aren't long-lasting like some other pain relief methods, this also means you can feel 'back to normal' quite quickly. You can walk around while using gas and air and use it in the birthing pool.

Labouring in water

Like the idea of floating your labour pains away in a pool? Water births are becoming increasingly common and popular as it's considered a natural way to keep relaxed and calm during labour.

During a water birth, you will be in a shallow tub or pool of warm water and supervised by a midwife. You may find it less restricting than being in a hospital bed and as birthing pools are wider and deeper than standard baths you can move around while keeping your bump immersed in water. Many women find it helps them to feel more in control. Plus, there's less pressure on your joints, helping you to feel lighter and more relaxed. The warm water can help you to feel calm, as well as easing your labour pains naturally. The disdvantage is that you'll only be able to use a birthing pool if your labour is considered 'low-risk' by your midwife. Unfortunately, there is also no guarantee that a birthing pool will be available if you do decide you want to have a water birth, as the majority of hospitals only have one pool. If you want to use one, let your midwife know when you discuss your birth plan and before you head to the hospital so he or she can see if one is available. If you opt for a home birth you can hire a pool.

Hypnotherapy

The use of hypnotherapy during labour has grown massively in the last few years. So much so that some hospitals are now offering it as a part of their antenatal classes.

It works by teaching you (and your birth partner) self-hypnosis techniques to help you feel calm during labour. You're encouraged to use positive language that moves away from the very medicalized words that are traditionally used during labour. For example, a contraction is known as a 'surge' or 'wave' and pain is called 'pressure' or 'tightening'.

You can either do an antenatal course on hypnobirthing (some run for a few hours a week over a few weeks, others are one- or two-day intensive courses), or you get a CD to listen to in the weeks leading up to the birth. Even if you plan on using pain-relief drugs during your labour, learning hypnobirthing techniques can still be useful as it will keep you calm throughout (especially if your circumstances change during labour and you need intervention). It is important to practise your relaxation and visualization techniques in the run up to your due date. Turn to page 75 for more on hypnobirthing.

Turn to page 75 for more on hypnobirthing.

EXPERT TIP

TEAM HYPNOBIRTH

Hypnobirthing is for couples, not just mothers. While you do the relaxing, your partner does everything else. You focus on your body and breathing and your partner keeps the room nice, talks to the midwives and plays the relaxing music. This way you can switch off into your relaxation and 'birthing mind-set'. Hypnobirthing also gives birth partners a clear role so they don't feel like a spare part.

When you do a hypnobirthing course, you will be sent home with a book and some hypnotic relaxation MP3s to listen to regularly. You will learn specific breathing techniques to use during your contractions, and some ideas of visualizations and affirmations to increase your relaxation and confidence. You will be asked to practise these every day until you go into labour. That way when you are in labour, you will find it much easier to stay physically and mentally relaxed, which will make for a less painful birth, and a quicker labour.

Mia Scotland
Doula

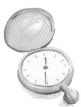

REAL LIFE

'Pethidine helped get me through labour'

'I'd been slightly suspicious of pethidine as a method of pain relief as I'd heard it could make your baby drowsy, but my antenatal teacher told me that timing was key, and that if you have it at the right point in your labour, it could really help. So I put it into my birth plan. When I went into labour, my cervix was taking a long time to dilate and I wasn't coping with the pain very well. I wanted an epidural, but when my midwife suggested trying pethidine first (and having an epidural afterwards if I still wasn't coping), I agreed. My contractions were still there, but they were less painful and meant I could rest. By the time I was ready to push, the pethidine had worn off, but I felt energized enough to deliver my baby. By the time Sunaina arrived she was bright-eyed and alert and started feeding straight away.'

BHAMINI, MUM TO SUNAINA,
14 MONTHS

Pethidine

An injection of pethidine isn't for everyone, but this strong painkiller may help you deal with contractions. The drug is a muscle relaxant and sedative, so if you're feeling very stressed and not coping with contractions, a shot of pethidine can help you. However, it doesn't have the same numbing effect as an epidural, so it's good if you want to keep moving around. It can also help to soften the cervix, so it can be useful if you've not been dilating.

The injection can be given by a midwife, and is usually administered in the top of your thigh or bottom. It takes about 20 minutes to kick in and can stay in the system for between two to four hours. However, the drug can cross the placenta and make your baby drowsy. It is not recommended if you are in the later stages of labour as it could make your baby sleepy when he's born and affect his sucking reflex, which could mean he's reluctant to feed.

Some women feel nauseous and dizzy after having pethidine and don't enjoy the feeling of being 'removed' and 'out of it', while other women find this sensation helps them doze a bit and gather their energy for the pushing stage.

Epidural

If you're really struggling with labour pain, or just want to be relatively pain free during labour and delivery, an epidural may be the best option for you. A local anaesthetic is injected into your spine and then a hollow needle is inserted, through which a tube is passed. The tube goes into the small of your back near your spinal column to deliver drugs that leave you numb from your stomach to your toes, effectively blocking out all the pain caused by your contractions.

You will need to be in a hospital in order to get an epidural, so if you plan to give birth at home or in a birth centre, you'll need to move. An epidural has to be administered by an anaesthetist and bear in mind that they are very busy. It can take some time for him or her to make their way round to you, so think about requesting early if you're planning on having one. You'll need to be in established labour with regular contractions before you can have one – and usually around 5cm (2 in) dilated.

Once your epidural has been set up, it can be topped up when needed, either by your midwife or often by you by clicking a button. Once you're fully dilated, your midwife will need to tell you when to start pushing as you won't feel the contractions. She does this by attaching a monitor to your stomach and watching for when a contraction is building.

Some women aim to let the epidural wear off a little as they're nearing the time to push so that they can then feel their contractions and know when to push. While lots of women choose to have epidurals, they are, in fact, just one version of a spinal anaesthesia. The other option is a spinal block. It's administered in the same way as an epidural, with anaesthetic medicine injected into fluid surrounding the spinal cord. The difference is that this is done without a catheter tube being inserted. It still numbs the body below the site of the injection

DID YOU KNOW?

Mums-to-be are much less likely to need an epidural or spinal block if they use a pool, tub or bath during the first stage of labour, according to studies.

but tends to be used for planned c-sections as the anaesthetist can administer the right amount of drug without having to give a top-up which you would have with an epidural.

CHAPTER TWELVE
STAGES OF LABOUR

It's been nine long months of waiting and preparing, but finally, the day has arrived that you feel those first genuine pangs of labour. Life is about to get very interesting, but before then, you've got labour and birth to get through. We've got news for you too, in most cases, babies like to take their time when making their arrival. Labour is a marathon, not a sprint. But if you know what to expect and are prepared and informed, you'll be able to get through it.

TAKING YOUR TIME

Labour is made up of three stages, and each stage can last differing amounts of time, depending on the woman. However, certain factors have been known to affect your length of labour, including whether this is your first or second baby, whether you've kept upright and active during labour, the strength of your contractions, having an epidural, the position of your baby and your general outlook.

Optimal foetal positioning: how is your baby lying?

The position of your baby within your pelvis as you near the end of your pregnancy can have an influence on your labour and the way your baby may be born. A baby that is in a favourable position before labour is said to be in an optimal foetal position. In an ideal world, your baby would lie head down, facing your back with her head either slightly turned to her left or right. This is known as 'occiput anterior' or OA.

However, babies don't always do what you want them to do (good preparation for life!) and occasionally she is either facing completely the wrong way, with her head facing up (known as a breech baby), or is facing down, but has her back facing your back, and her tummy facing your tummy. This is known as 'occiput posterior' or OP. A baby in the OP position can cause a strong back ache when you go into labour, and labours tend to take longer as she has to twist round in order to be born. While you can't force your baby to lie in a certain position, there are exercises (see above) that you can do from 28 weeks of pregnancy to encourage your baby to move into an OA position.

1

FIRST STAGE OF LABOUR

This is generally the longest stage of labour as it's when your cervix is thinning ready for delivery. While you may have been having contractions for a while, the early part is known as the latent phase, or pre-labour and early labour. Many midwives don't count the first stage of labour as having really begun until you're around 3–4cm (1¼–1½in) dilated and contractions are well established. This goes some way to explaining why many mums talk about having a three-day labour. While statistics suggest that the average labour lasts about 12 to 18 hours it totally depends on when you count it as having started; was it with the early twinges or when you're having regular contractions?

Your early contractions may feel like period pains, but as they build they'll last longer and feel much stronger. Try to stay as active as possible during this stage. Most women find they are more comfortable staying at home for a few hours, but it's best to call the hospital or your midwife who can advise the best course of action.

Once you arrive at hospital, your midwife will give you an internal examination to check how dilated your cervix is – once you're 4cm (1½in) or more you're in 'active labour' and will be taken to the delivery room to have your baby. You should start thinking about your pain relief options now (see chapter 11, pages 110–15) and decide if you need anything straight away or whether you want to hold off for now.

Boost your labour energy levels

Give yourself an extra injection of energy during labour with these four quick tips:

● **Stay hydrated**. Drink plenty of water, regular sips are ideal. If you're struggling to eat, but you feel like you could stomach a fizzy drink, an energy drink can help you through some tiring contractions.

● **Be a savvy snacker.** Carbohydrates are good to eat during labour as they're easily digested and give a slow release of energy – and will help you through contractions. If you can stomach it, try snacking on wholemeal sandwiches or pasta salads. Eat little and often, rather than having one big meal. Snack on oatcakes, banana and nuts to fill you up and keep you going.

● **Keep your birth partner going.** Whether it's your husband, mum or friend holding your hand through labour, it's worth remembering that your birth partner will need to keep their energy levels up too. Labour can be long and tiring for them, so encourage them to take regular food and drink breaks.

● **Pace yourself.** Once you get to 10cm (4in) dilated, your baby still has to make her way down the birth canal. Don't start pushing right away, or you might run out of steam – wait until you get the urge. When you feel you want to start, listen to your midwife and she'll coach you through it.

HAVING AN INTERNAL EXAMINATION

In order for your midwife to assess what stage you're at in your labour, you'll need to have an internal examination. The midwife will put on gloves and, often after using an antiseptic obstetric cream, he or she will insert their fingers into your vagina to measure whether your cervix has started dilating. The muscles in your uterus contract in order to open your cervix, making it thinner and softer in order to allow your baby to pass through.

Each midwife will have their own way of measuring how dilated you are, although it's often based on how many fingers they can fit through the cervix, or whether they can feel any cervix at all. Obviously, people have different sized fingers (and if you have a male midwife, his hands and fingers will usually be bigger), which is why they will have worked out their own system of measuring how far along you are.

There's no getting away from the fact that these internal exams can be uncomfortable, and for some women, very painful. If this is the case, let your midwife know so she can take her time, but the key is to relax (not easy when you're having contractions). Rather like when you have a smear test, if you tense up, it will make the whole procedure more painful.

You are most likely to be examined around every four hours while you're in labour, but this will depend on the length of your labour. If you really can't bear having an internal examination, you do have the right to refuse. While this can make a midwife's job a little trickier, particularly when advising you on whether you should have a particular type of pain relief, there are other signs she can look for to inform her on how your labour is progressing.

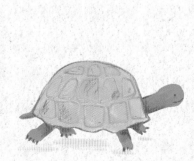

FINDING THE RIGHT BIRTH POSITION

If there's one thing that all midwives and obstetricians will recommend, is that you try and stay as active as possible during labour. We're not talking about star jumps and lunges between contractions, but finding positions that are comfortable for you, that can also aid labour will help you in the long run. It might be worth practising a few of these positions with your birth partner before the big day, but whatever happens, be open to change and suggestions.

Leaning forward
Stand with your knees bent and lean forward over a bed, chair or sofa, to get labour going in the early stages. This position uses gravity to help your baby move down towards the cervix. You may get tired quite quickly, though, so alternate with sitting positions.

Walking
Nothing happening? Pace through your house or around the hospital ward. Moving around during early labour encourages your baby's head to move down and, as an added bonus, it may take your mind off the pain of your contractions. However, if your baby needs to be monitored or you have an epidural, this will restrict how far you can walk or if you can walk at all.

The standing hug
Much like walking, this uses gravity to help your baby along, but you stay still in a hugging position with your birth partner. He or she will need to be strong enough to support you as you lean forward (so try doing this with your partner leaning against a wall for support). This is also a great way to feel close and supported during labour.

Sitting
Sit on a birth ball with your knees apart or sit back-to-front on a chair with no arms. Tilt forward so your tummy is between your knees. You're still working with gravity to help things along, but this position also allows you to relax between contractions.

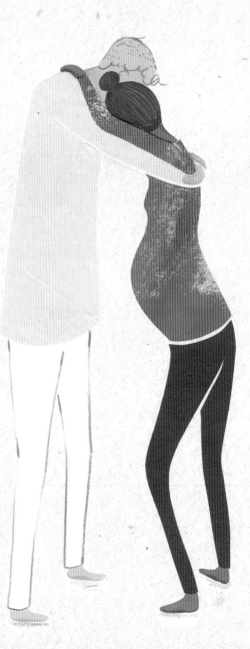

Squatting

When it comes to the second stage of labour (the pushing part), get on your haunches with your partner sitting on a chair behind you. Rest your back against your partner's legs, with your arms along his thighs. You're less likely to have a tear in this position, as it gives your baby more space to arrive.

All fours

Kneeling on a mat or on a bed, go into an all-fours position. You can either rest on your hands or, if that's too tiring, lean down onto your elbows between contractions. This is a great position for pushing out your baby. Your pelvis will be open and gravity will be able to propel delivery. This should make the pushing stage shorter and less painful for you. It's also a great position for getting your partner to massage your back. Your knees may start to ache after a while, so rest on a yoga mat.

Kneeling

Get on the floor and spread your knees hip-width apart, then lean over a birth ball or bed. While this may really ease the pressure for you, it's a difficult position for a midwife to see what's going on, so you may have to move into all fours at the end.

APPROACHING THE SECOND STAGE

It is common for women to switch off and lose focus of their surroundings while labouring. If this happens to you it is a great sign as it means you're letting your natural instincts and your body take over to birth your baby.

Your baby's head is starting to descend now, so you might even feel like you're going to do a poo but don't worry, this is normal and is actually a good sign. You might also feel the urge to push, but try not to as it's still too early as you're still not fully dilated.

At the end of the first stage of labour you'll be fully dilated (10cm/4in) and may start feeling an urge to push. Let your midwife know and she will guide you through the next stage.

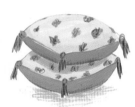

REAL LIFE

'All fours worked for me'

'I'd practised various positions for birth during my antenatal classes, but didn't really know what would work best until I was in labour. I was having a home birth, so was really keen to try as many of them as possible. I started out propped up in a nest of cushions, and alternated this with leaning over my bed. As my labour progressed, I could tell I was getting more tired, but I still wanted a position that felt like I was helping my baby along. My midwife suggested going on all fours, with cushions under my knees. It really helped and I ended up pushing my baby out in that position, with the midwife catching my baby between my legs.'

KERRY, MUM TO JORDAN, TWO, AND MILLIE, THREE

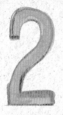

SECOND STAGE OF LABOUR

The second stage of your labour usually lasts between one and two hours, but this can vary from woman to woman, and often depends on whether this is your first or second baby. If you feel like you need to push, tell your midwife. It's important she can ensure you're fully dilated first, as doing it prematurely can increase the risk of tearing your cervix.

Once you're fully dilated, your baby will move down the birth canal. It may feel at this point like your body is taking over, and this is perfectly normal. Just go with it as your body instinctively knows what to do. Contractions may seem shorter, with a greater lull between them, so your midwife will be monitoring them and coaching you to push down when each one happens. Try to keep breathing while pushing. Holding your breath will just make you and your baby more tired as you'll be reducing the amount of oxygen getting to your muscles.

Eventually your baby's head will crown, which is when it starts to come through the opening to your vagina; and you can even reach down and touch it – or see it if you have a mirror. As your baby's head is born, you may feel a stinging sensation. It's important that you listen to your midwife carefully, as she'll probably tell you to stop pushing or just push gently and breathe using short pants at this point. This is to stop you from tearing the perineum – the area between your vagina and anus.

Once the head is out, your baby will twist round to allow the shoulders to be born – with help from your midwife – and the rest of the body will slip out. Your midwife will dry the baby, rubbing the skin quite vigorously to encourage circulation and your baby to breathe on her own. She'll place the baby on your chest (if that's what you've agreed) and you'll get your first look at your newborn and you can cuddle her for the first time. Skin-to-skin contact now will help you establish a bond with your baby. You midwife will soon weigh and measure your baby and check her over carefully.

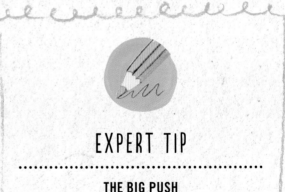

EXPERT TIP

....

THE BIG PUSH

The urge to push or bear down is a strong instinctive feeling which is hard to miss! Follow your body's guidance, but if you do find it difficult, your midwife will be there to support and guide you with the pushing. Sometimes it takes a few contractions before your pushing becomes effective — this is quite normal.

Helen Taylor
Midwife

3

THIRD STAGE OF LABOUR

Even though you'll be holding your precious bundle in your arms by now, labour's not quite over yet. Your baby is still attached to your placenta via the umbilical cord. There's a growing trend for midwives and obstetricians to hold off clamping and cutting the cord for at least two minutes after birth until the blood flow to the placenta stops. Studies have found that doing so has extra health benefits to your baby, including improved antioxidant capacity and a reduced inflammatory response from the birth. Both aid development in your newborn in the first few days after birth.

Once the cord is clamped, either the midwife (or your birth partner if he or she wishes) can cut the umbilical cord, which is then fixed with a clip and will eventually dry up and drop off.

Now it's time to deliver the placenta. You might feel contractions as this happens, and they can be quite powerful but don't worry, this is normal. It's also common to feel shaky because of the change in body temperature and loss of fluid, as well as the sheer effort of childbirth. Delivering the placenta can take anything from five minutes to an hour and many women are given a syntocinon injection to speed up the process. It works by stimulating the uterus to contract, expelling the placenta and preventing any further bleeding. If you wish to deliver the placenta without drugs, let your midwife know. Once the placenta has been delivered, you'll be wheeled into the postnatal ward so you can spend time with your baby.

Q&A

'I don't want the cord cut immediately – how can I ensure this happens?'

Midwife **HELEN TAYLOR** says, 'Increasing research has found that holding off cutting the umbilical cord for a few minutes can be beneficial for your baby's health. If you want to ensure that the midwives hold off clamping the cord, put it in your birth plan, but also make sure your birth partner knows your wishes so he or she can ensure that this happens. It's easy to be distracted by the arrival of your baby, so if there's someone there to remind people, that will help.'

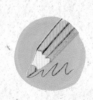

EXPERT TIP

THE BENEFIT OF SUCKLING

In addition to the injection used to help the womb contract and deliver the placenta, your baby suckling from your breast also gives your body a surge of oxytocin, which helps the womb to contract.

Shreelata Datta
Obstetrician

THE BIRTH

The first stage is in several phases: the latent – which includes pre-labour and early labour – then established or active labour, which begins when you are 3cm (1¼in) dilated. Your midwife can assess how far along you are with an internal examination around every four hours, depending on the length of your labour. You do have a right to refuse this, but it can make the midwife's job a little trickier and she can't tell you how far along you are.

STAGE 1

Your uterus is very heavy now and you'll probably be feeling uncomfortable and ready to meet your baby. You may be experiencing 'false labour' or Braxton Hicks contractions. If you are overdue you might be given the offer of being induced to speed things along.

STARTING OFF

At over 3cm (1¼in) dilated you're officially in active labour – it's important to keep your energy levels up with carbohydrate snacks. This is the time to go to hospital if you are not there already.

ACTIVE LABOUR

STAY ACTIVE

Try to stay active and find which labour position is most comfortable. Remember to pace yourself and don't start pushing until your midwife says you are ready.

CONTRACTIONS

Early contractions may feel a bit like period pains – they will build up and become stronger and longer. They are gradually making your cervix open up and 'efface'.

THIRD STAGE

The third stage is cutting the umbilical cord and delivery of the placenta – you might still feel contractions and this stage can take anywhere between five minutes and an hour, though it can be sped up with a syntocinon injection.

As you move from the first to the second stage of labour you may have a strong urge to push – this is known as transition.

TRANSITION

You may feel a burning sensation as baby's head crowns.

CROWNING

STAGE 2

The midwife may ask you to push slowly so you don't tear and he is not delivered too quickly.

DELIVERY

STAGE 3

SECOND STAGE

Your midwife will check that you're fully dilated and then you can start pushing with each contraction. Try to keep breathing while pushing and listen to the midwife when she tells you to push more gently.

YOUR BABY!

After the baby is born the midwife will dry him vigorously to encourage circulation and you'll get to meet your little one!

CHAPTER THIRTEEN
BIRTH OUTCOMES AND INTERVENTIONS

In an ideal world, every birth would be completely hiccup-free, and the only help you need would be from your midwife as you deliver your baby. However, the reality is different, and so it's important you're prepared and informed in case you do need some kind of medical intervention during the birth.

TEARING CAN HAPPEN

The pressure of your baby pushing down can create small tears in the opening to the vagina and the perineum, the area between the vagina and the anus. Tearing is not uncommon, but the tears usually heal quickly and do not always need stitches. They are usually classified as first-, second-, third- or fourth-degree tears. First-degree tears affect the skin of the perineum and the back of the vagina. They're often small and don't need stitching. A tear is second degree if the muscles of the perineum are torn as well. If the the anal sphincter muscle is also partially or completely torn, this is a third-degree injury. A tear is described as fourth degree if the damage extends into the rectum as well. Second-, third- and fourth-degree tears will need to be repaired by your midwife or an obstetrician after the birth.

Once your baby is born the midwife will inspect the area. Your legs will be put in stirrups, the perineal area will be cleaned with antiseptic and numbed with a local anaesthetic so you won't feel anything. Any soreness or discomfort can be relieved using painkillers such as paracetamol. The stitches are made using dissolvable thread, so you won't need to have them removed. Your midwife will check that the area is healing when he or she visits you at home.

DID YOU KNOW?

Nine out of ten mums tear to some extent during childbirth, but a third of those won't need any treatment and the tears heal on their own.

QUICK FIX

A GENTLE MASSAGE

Massaging your perineum during pregnancy can make it more flexible for birth, which helps prevent tearing. Gently massage and stretch the skin around your perineum using an unperfumed oil. Insert your finger or thumb (or get your partner to do it) about 2cm (1in) into your vagina and knead and stretch the opening. Do this for a few minutes each day.

WHAT IS AN EPISIOTOMY?

Sometimes your midwife or obstetrician will make a cut in your perineum (the area between your vagina and anus) to make the opening of your vagina wider. This is called an episiotomy. While there probably isn't one mum-to-be who would choose to have one, they can help your labour along – especially if you're overtired, your baby needs a helping hand arriving using forceps or a ventouse or it looks like your baby needs more space to be delivered because he has a large head.

Episiotomies are only performed if necessary during delivery and it can be hard to predict whether it's needed until the second stage of labour. The cut will be made large enough for your baby to fit through, but will be done with extreme precision to not damage anything permanently.

You will need to lie down on the bed with your feet in stirrups. Your perineum will be cleaned with antiseptic and numbed with a local anaesthetic. If you've already had an epidural, this may be topped up to completely deaden the area. Either way, you won't feel a thing. If you do, tell your midwife. He or she will make a cut at a slight angle using a pair of special scissors or a scalpel. Don't be surprised if your baby is born almost immediately afterwards – this is normal.

Once your baby has arrived, you'll be stitched up with a dissolvable thread. This takes around 30 minutes, but you'll probably be completely preoccupied by your baby and will barely notice what's going on down there. You should feel back to normal within about six weeks of giving birth, as the perineum tends to heal quickly. It's very rare that you'll need anything re-stitched, but if you do then your midwife will advise.

EXPERT TIP

YOUR BIRTH, YOUR CHOICE

The National Institute for Health & Clinical Excellence (NICE) guidelines say a pregnant woman can request a Caesarean delivery for a reason that isn't necessarily medical, such as fear of labour (tocophobia). Counselling will be offered on the pros and cons of a Caesarean versus vaginal birth. It is important to consider the consequences for future pregnancies and the benefit of labour for your baby's lungs. If you want a Caesarean and your hospital can't book you one, you can ask to be referred elswhere.

Shreelata Datta
Obstetrician

FORCEPS AND VENTOUSE BIRTHS

Sometimes your baby needs help during the pushing stage and your obstetrician may use forceps or a ventouse to help deliver him – this is known as an assisted delivery.

Forceps look like large metal salad tongs. They come apart separately, but can clip together. They're designed to fit around your baby's head and cradle it, not squash it. A ventouse is a small cup that fits on the back of your baby's head and is attached to a suction device. A vacuum is created using either a hand-held pump or via electricity so that your doctor can then gently pull your baby out during your contraction. Before applying either, you will be given some local anaesthetic unless you've already had an epidural.

Deciding which method to use

The decision as to whether your obstetrician uses a ventouse or forceps depends on each birth. You may deliver in a labour room or be taken to the operating theatre, as if it fails then the doctor can perform a Caesarean section (see page 130). Forceps are often used if the baby needs to be born quickly or if you are finding it difficult to push, as they're a much faster method of delivery. However, they may cause vaginal tears and leave marks on your baby's face (although these fade in a few days). A ventouse is often the first option as there's less risk of tearing, but it has a lower chance of success. If that doesn't work, the obstetrician may move on to forceps. A ventouse can leave a bruise on your baby's head, which usually fades within 48 hours. An episiotomy (see page 127) is more likely to be considered during a forceps delivery as extra room is needed to guide each of the blades around your baby's head. You need to be fully dilated and the head needs to be at the opening of the cervix.

Your pain relief

If you haven't already had an epidural, you will be given some form of pain relief before the ventouse or forceps are inserted. This could be through an epidural or a pudendal block (where an anaesthetic is injected into a nerve in your vaginal wall to numb any pain in that area). If the birthing team have to deliver your baby quickly, there may not be time for an anaesthetist to administer an epidural, and a pudendal block will be faster.

How a ventouse works

After assessing the position of your baby's head, the obstetrician will fit the ventouse cap to the back of the head and turn on the suction. When you have a contraction, he'll start pulling on the ventouse to ease your baby out. He can't pull too hard otherwise he'll lose the suction, but he may have to perform an episiotomy to assist the delivery. Your baby may have a small bump on his head where the ventouse was attached. This is known as a chignon, and it's caused by the suction drawing the baby's scalp up. Don't worry too much as the bump will start to go down within half an hour. There may also be a small bruise on his head, again this will disappear after a day or two.

How a forceps delivery is performed

After assessing the position of your baby's head, the obstetrician will slide first one part of the forceps, then the other so that they cradle the baby's head, and he or she will clip them together. When you have your next contraction, he'll ask you to push while he pulls. As your baby's head is crowning, the obstetrician may need to perform an episiotomy (see page 127). This isn't always necessary and may not happen, but does in the majority of cases, as it helps your baby's head be born. Your baby may have red marks on his face from the forceps, but these should disappear after a couple of days. Forceps have a higher

success rate when delivering babies than the ventouse. However, if your baby isn't born after three contractions and pulls, the forceps will be abandoned and a Caesarean delivery may be necessary (see page 130).

Q&A

I've heard having a forceps delivery can ruin your pelvic floor muscles. Is this true?

Obstetrician **SHREELATA DATTA** says, 'Your pelvic floor forms a broad sling of muscles, ligaments and supportive tissues that stretch from your pubic bone at the front of your body, to the base of your spine at the back. Whilst they are able to stretch down, the muscles and tissues can be weakened if they bear weight for a long time, as in pregnancy. In addition, pushing for a long time, delivering a large baby, sustaining a large vaginal tear and a forceps delivery can weaken them. So it's really important to start pelvic floor exercises as early 32 weeks into pregnancy and continue for at least the first three months after your baby is born. This minimizes the risk of long-term urinary incontinence and keeps the pelvic floor muscles strong. Every time you become pregnant, the muscles of your pelvic floor stretch and delivery by Caesarean cannot reverse the pressure and weight on your pelvic floor from the previous months.'

WHAT IS A CAESAREAN SECTION?

With one in four babies born by Caesarean, also know as a C-section, it's important to understand why one might be necessary. It's thought around half of all Caesareans are elective, mostly because of a known likelihood of complications during the birth. The rest are emergency, which means the birth is not going to plan and a complication has developed with either the mother or the baby. The former doesn't necessarily mean that you're 'too posh to push'. It simply means that the operation has been planned in advance.

Medical considerations

For most women, a vaginal birth is the ideal way to bring their baby into the world but, for some, medical reasons means a C-section is the safer option for both the mother and the baby. Possible reasons include placenta praevia, in which a low-lying placenta is completely or partially blocking the baby's exit route, or a breech presentation, where the baby is lying feet or bottom first. A vaginal birth is sometimes possible for these situations, so you'll be referred to your obstetrician for a review. But you should be prepared that a C-section is on the cards. A C-section is likely to be recommended if you are expecting twins.

Urgent attention

Giving birth doesn't always go to plan and, occasionally, an emergency C-section may be your only option. Knowing what to expect will help you through it, so prepare for every eventuality. It may not be as rushed and stressful as it sounds, depending on the reason why you need to have one. It's simply unplanned and carried out when complications occur after natural labour has started. It could be because

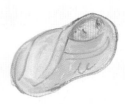

REAL LIFE

'I needed an emergency Caesarean'

'After arriving at hospital with my contractions two minutes apart, I was disappointed to discover I was only 3cm (1¼in) dilated. But a few hours in the birthing pool with some gas and air and I was astonished to discover I was nearly 8cm (3¼in) dilated. I asked for an epidural as the pain was intense and was pleased to start pushing a few hours later. Unfortunately, Layla did not want to come out and after pushing for nearly two hours, the doctor explained they weren't happy with her progress and they'd detected meconium (a baby's first bowel movement, which can signal distress). They said it would be safer to go for an emergency Caesarean. I was wheeled into theatre and about ten minutes later Layla was born. It wasn't the birth I'd planned, but it was what was right at the time, and the most important thing was that she arrived safely.'

HELEN, MUM TO LAYLA, FOUR MONTHS

things aren't progressing as they should. The baby may be lying in an awkward position, you may be struggling or your baby may have become distressed.

How it's done

You'll be given an epidural or spinal block (if you haven't already had one), which allows you to stay awake during the procedure. Occasionally you may need a general anaesthetic. You'll be wheeled into the operating theatre and a fabric screen will be placed over your abdomen to reduce the risk of infection – and another one may be placed in front of your head so you can't see what is going on. You'll be allowed one birth partner in with you, and he or she will be encouraged to sit by your head. An incision is made just above your pubic hairline, through the abdominal wall to your uterus. You may feel a strange tugging sensation, especially as the baby is delivered, but you shouldn't feel any pain. It takes about ten minutes from first incision to deliver your baby. You'll be shown your baby, who'll then be cleaned up, wrapped in a blanket and handed to you and your partner. The obstetrician will then deliver the placenta, make sure your womb has contracted and check that your ovaries look healthy before stitching your womb and skin in layers; your scar will be 10–15cm (4–6in) long. The whole operation usually takes 40 minutes and afterwards you (and your baby) will be taken to a recovery room for monitoring.

If you do end up having a Caesarean, you'll be left with a small line where your pubic hair begins. It's usually a few inches long and will be covered in a dressing initially. This can be removed a couple of days after the birth. You'll need to be careful when holding your baby as you don't want to risk splitting the wound, and it's why doctors advise against lifting your baby (or any other heavy item) or driving. You need to keep the area as clean and dry as possible, looking out for any redness or discharge as it could be a sign of an infection. The scar will appear very red at first.

It will eventually fade, but that could take a few months – sometimes longer. A couple of years after the birth, it will have faded to a faint line, but this depends on your skin tone – for people who have light skin tones, it will fade to a silvery line, those with darker skin tones may find it stays darker and may appear more raised.

Recovery time

The procedure is relatively straightforward but it is major abdominal surgery. You'll be kept in hospital for a few days to check you're healing and then you'll be allowed home. Your community midwife will check that your scar is healing on her home visits. You'll still experience vaginal bleeding after the delivery, although this usually resolves within six weeks. Most stitches are made using dissolvable thread so you probably won't need them removed, but if not, your midwife will remove them seven to ten days later.

Heavy lifting and driving are off limits for the first six weeks, and you should avoid any exercise for 12 weeks, or certainly until you've had the all clear from your doctor.

QUICK FIX

SCAR HEALING

Try rubbing vitamin E oil into your skin (only when it's fully healed) to help the scar fade faster. It promotes the development of collagen fibres in the skin, which are needed for soft tissue healing.

CHAPTER FOURTEEN
AFTER THE BIRTH

Congratulations! You've become a mum! The next 24 hours will probably whizz by in a blur of feeding, first nappy changes, phone calls and texts, sleep (hopefully) and proud glances at your little bundle. But this is also a really important time for you and your baby, as it's when you'll start bonding with your newborn, feeding him and recovering from birth.

BONDING WITH YOUR NEWBORN

When your baby is first born, she may be given a quick wipe down to remove any amniotic fluid. Your midwife will try not to remove too much of the vernix – the waxy substance that covers your baby – as it protects her skin in the first days. She will usually be placed straight onto your chest for a cuddle, some special skin-to-skin contact and her first feed, so the bonding process that you began during pregnancy can continue. She may spend around 20 minutes looking about, adjusting to her new environment. All babies are different though, so she may fall asleep or start 'rooting' for your breast. Some babies latch on immediately, others need guidance; your midwife will help. After your baby has had skin-to-skin contact and a feed, your midwife will put her in a nappy.

You may notice that your baby is already trying to focus on you. When she is born she can see about 20–30cm (10–12in) in front of her, just far enough to be able to make eye contact with you when you hold her. Her eyesight takes around six months to establish, but in the meantime she'll be fascinated by very simple and contrasting patterns. Researchers at Stanford University, USA, have discovered that a baby can make out a face at just an hour old. It's thought this is an instinct that helps with bonding.

When you talk to her, you may be amazed at how she calms down and stops crying. That's because she's soothed by the sound of your voice as she recognizes it from when she was in the womb.

The bonding process can take a while to kick in. It's very normal to not feel an immediate connection with your baby; don't worry, as it will appear when you least expect it. If you had a traumatic labour, your baby has a health problem or you're exhausted, you may not feel a bond straight away.

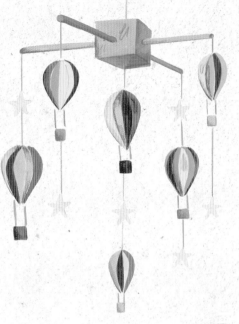

Q&A

'Why is skin-to-skin time important after the birth?'

Midwife **HELEN TAYLOR** says, 'Skin-to-skin time is important as it helps with bonding. Your baby gets to know you through touch and smell and placing her on your chest will mean she's next to your skin and can smell your unique natural scent. It can also encourage breastfeeding. Your midwife may suggest putting your baby skin-to-skin on your chest straight after birth. Once delivered and placed onto your chest, the midwife will wipe your baby with a dry towel, then leave her on your chest with a clean towel placed over you both.

FEEDING YOUR BABY

During pregnancy, your baby was laying down reserves of fat under the skin to provide energy for her in the first few days of life. That's because it can take two or three days for your proper breast milk to 'come in' – that is, be available for feeding. Until then, you can still breastfeed your baby as your breasts are producing a nutrient and antibody-rich substance called colostrum, but the real food won't begin for a few days. Plus, if you breastfeed now, you can get help on making sure your baby is latching on correctly.

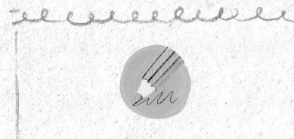

EXPERT TIP

GETTING A GOOD LATCH WITH YOUR BABY

The key to breastfeeding is a good latch and having a base knowledge about achieving that latch is ideal so read up about it beforehand or attend a teaching session in pregnancy. Once your baby is born, get as much support as you can from midwifery staff. Encourage your baby to open his mouth as wide as possible so he can fit as much of the nipple and breast in as he can. The tongue, bottom lip and chin should touch the breast first and your baby's nose should be free so he can breathe properly.

Helen Taylor
Midwife

You'll know when your breast milk comes in because your breasts will become engorged, hard and almost painful. Breastfeeding will help to relieve this, but also make sure you wear a supportive breastfeeding bra.

BEFORE YOU GO HOME

The time you spend in hospital or your birth centre will vary depending on your birth. Some mums can go home a few hours after birth, while others will need to stay overnight or for a few days. Before you go you and the baby will be checked by a midwife, and a child health doctor – a paediatrician – will examine your baby too.

Checking you after the birth

Your midwife will carry out a postnatal check. This will include checking your tummy and making sure that the uterus is beginning to contract, and to check your bleeding. You will bleed for around four to six weeks after birth, which is known as lochia. He or she will also check if you've got a good latch for breastfeeding, and help you with that if not. If you need pain relief for stitches, she can provide some and advise on what you can have once you're at home.

Checking your baby

Straight after the birth your midwife will carry out checks on your newborn. He or she will measure her weight and length, temperature, and the circumference of her head. Before you leave the hospital a paediatrician will carry out a full newborn check looking at all areas of her body. He or she will check her heartbeat, breathing pattern, eyesight, hearing, hands, feet, spine, hips and reflex movements. He or she will also arrange for a hearing screening. If you baby is born at home your midwife will do this.

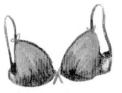

REAL LIFE

....

'My breasts felt like rocks'

'After my son was born, I was keen to breastfeed as I figured it was the easiest way to feed him. For the first few days, I managed to get a good latch and give him colostrum. He didn't feed for long, but the midwife said he only needed small amounts at this stage. A couple of days after I got home, my breasts started to feel hot and achey. They felt like rocks and I knew my milk had come in. Breastfeeding eased it, but I also tried hand expressing some of the milk. A day or two after this, my breasts started feeling fine, so long as I fed regularly.'

ANNIE, MUM TO PATRICK, THREE,
AND SARAH, ONE

Ready to go

Once it's time to go, make sure you dress yourself and your baby in warm, comfy clothing. You'll still need your maternity clothes as you'll have a sizeable bump, which will take a couple of weeks to go down. Your baby will need to be dressed in a vest, baby-gro and warm all-in-one suit and he'll also need a hat.

QUICK FIX

....

VISITORS

Having too many visitors in the early weeks after birth can be both exhausting and overwhelming. Instead, make sure you only receive visitors in twos and threes and book them in for set times to ensure it doesn't get too much. If you're very tired either ask your visitors to bring you a meal or put them off until you are feeling better.

EXPERT TIP

....

COPING WITH POST-BIRTH SORENESS

Taking arnica tablets could help to ease soreness and bruising associated with stitches. An inflatable ring can make sitting less uncomfortable and take the recommended dose of paracetamol if you're in pain. Avoid constipation by drinking plenty of water and eating a high-fibre diet. If you notice that any bleeding or discharge is smelly talk to your midwife as this could suggest an infection.

Shreelata Datta
Obstetrician

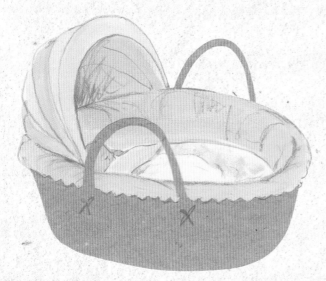

GOING HOME

If you haven't sorted your home out in preparation for your baby's arrival now, ask your partner, a friend or relative to make sure it's fully prepared for when you leave hospital. You will need:

- a Moses basket
- newborn babygros
- newborn nappies
- wipes
- feeding pillow
- breastfeeding clothes if you're breastfeeding
- breast pads
- a fully stocked fridge and freezer
- snacks to keep energy levels up

Adapting to your new life

Once you've got home, you will probably do what every new parent does. Look down at your baby and think, 'What on earth do I do now?!' It can be daunting, but if you look at the next few weeks as just a series of firsts, which you simply need to get through (and hopefully enjoy) one day at a time, then you'll be fine.

Baby's first poo

If your baby hasn't passed his first poo after birth or before leaving hospital, then this will be an interesting experience for you at home. The first poo is known as meconium, and is a green-black sticky substance very unlike normal baby poo. It can be difficult to clean off, but don't worry, once your baby starts drinking milk, it will change to a more yellow-brown runny poo.

Baby's first feed

You'll hopefully have had a successful attempt at feeding your baby while in hospital, but if you're breastfeeding, this is usually colostrum and your baby won't need much. Once your breast milk 'comes in' a few days later, feeding can take longer. While making sure you get a good latch (see page 134) is important, you should also ensure that you are totally comfortable while you feed. Whether laid up in bed with plenty of pillows or in a comfy chair, make sure you have everything you need to hand. This includes a glass of water as breastfeeding can be very dehydrating, snacks to keep energy levels up, a pillow or cushion to rest your baby on so that he's at the right height to feed and your arms don't start aching, and something to keep you occupied if it's going to be a long feed, such as a book or magazine.

Baby's first night at home

Because babies take a while to get the concept of night and day, and need feeding regularly, his first night at home will probably take on a similar pattern to his first day. He'll need to be fed on demand – usually every few hours – so be prepared to be up at all hours. And while the best advice is to try and sleep when your baby sleeps, that's not always the easiest thing, so don't beat yourself up if you don't manage that. Even being awake, but just resting will have a restorative effect on tired new mums. Just don't try to cram washing in the machine or make tea and biscuits for visitors while your baby is asleep! This is where *they* can help *you* by letting you put your feet up to rest.

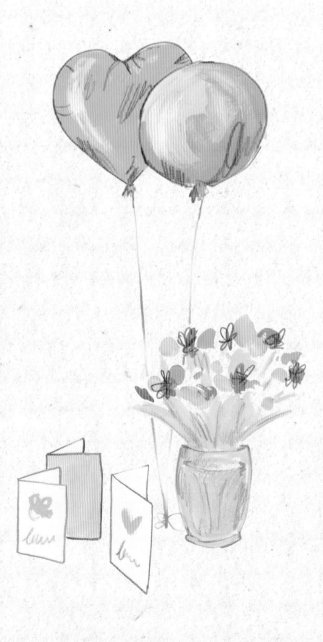

EXPERT TIP

SAFER SLEEPING FOR YOUR BABY

To reduce the risk of sudden infant death syndrome (SIDS), it's important to follow these guidlines. Always place your baby on her back to sleep, with her feet at the bottom of the cot so she can't slip under her blanket and overheat. Keep your baby away from cigarette smoke while you are pregnant and after birth. Make sure her cot or Moses basket has a firm flat new mattress and have her sleep in your room for the first six months. Keep the room she sleeps in at around 16–20°C (61–68°F). Use light bedding or a lightweight well-fitting baby sleep bag that is comfortable and safe for sleeping babies.

Don't sleep on a sofa or in an armchair with your baby or have her in your bed if you smoke, drink or take drugs or are extremely tired, if she was born prematurely or was of low birth-weight. Never allow her to become too hot. Never cover her face or head while she's sleeping.

Helen Taylor
Midwife

RECOVERY AND YOUR 6-WEEK CHECK-UP

You may think your little bundle just sleeps and feeds, but from day one she's soaking up information. She's already aware that her new surroundings – the outside world – are different from the womb, and she'll crave the environment she's enjoyed for the last nine months. She'll want to feel warm and safe so she'll probably just want to feed and be held a lot to begin with. Right from the beginning babies listen, watch and start to recognize people and objects, and from around the four- to six-week mark, you may get that magical first smile.

Learning your new way of life

For the next few weeks, you'll be getting to grips with looking after your baby and being a mum. Some things will come easily to you and others may be trickier, but as long as you have a great support network to fall back on, you'll be able to cope. You should get a visit from your community midwife once you're at home, and she'll check how you're coping and whether your baby is feeding well. It's normal for newborns to lose some of their body weight in the first week and then start putting on weight to reach and then surpass their birth weight. If this isn't the case, talk to your midwife to check your baby is eating enough.

EXPERT TIP

BABY BLUES V. POSTNATAL DEPRESSION

Look out for post-baby blues. A combination of exhaustion and still fluctuating hormones could see you feeling tearful for no apparent reason. If, however, you're still low at around six weeks, and the feeling is coupled with hopelessness, a lack of interest or even hostility towards your baby, dark thoughts and feeling like you can't cope, talk to your doctor, as it could be a sign of postnatal depression.

Dr Ellie Cannon
GP

QUICK FIX

COPING WITH BABY BRAIN

Write down any issues or questions for your doctor before your six-week check-up so you don't forget what you want to say or ask — easy when you're a tired new mum with lots on her mind. And if possible, take someone with you so he or she can look after the baby and you can get time with the doctor on your own and undistracted.

First development and health checks

At around six to eight weeks, you'll have some check-ups with your doctor. You'll be responsible for booking these check-ups, so think about booking in your appointment about two to three weeks after the birth so you don't forget. One check-up is designed to look at the health and development of your baby (and start her immunization) and the other is to see how you are doing. In your check-up, your doctor will:

- Ask if you're fully recovered from birth.

- Ask about your pelvic floor – whether you're passing water and opening your bowels as both can be affected by childbirth.

- Check if your bleeding (lochia) has stopped.

- Talk to you about sex and contraception and find out which method you'll be using now. If you use a cap he or she will need to check the size as your cervix will have changed.

- Check that you're comfortable with breastfeeding if that's how you've chosen to feed your baby.

- Look at your Caesarean scar if you had one and make sure it's healed well.

- Give you a smear test if it's due.

- Check your blood pressure.

- Talk to you about any medications that you might have been on before your pregnancy and whether they need to be restarted or changed back.

- Find out how you're coping emotionally and ensure you're happy. Your doctor will be looking specifically for signs of postnatal depression, so be honest about how you feel.

If everything is healing well and you feel happy in yourself, you'll only need to see your GP for your baby's regular vaccinations, or if either one of you is ill. If you're not feeling completely happy, don't be afraid to bring it up with your doctor, even if the only reason you're at the clinic is for your baby. Now is the time to share any issues you have.

Whether pregnancy has been a rollercoaster of ups and downs, or a walk in the park, we hope that you've enjoyed the experience. Your next adventure is just beginning... Good luck!

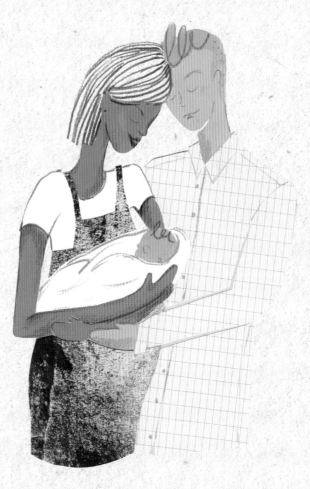

NOTES

CONGRATULATIONS ON YOUR LITTLE BUNDLE
OF JOY! USE THESE PAGES TO MAKE NOTES
ON YOUR PREGNANCY JOURNEY AND PLAN
THE EXCITING MONTHS AHEAD.

NOTES

NOTES

NOTES

NOTES

NOTES

GLOSSARY

Active birth Where a pregnant woman is encouraged to move around as much as possible during labour, taking different positions, rather than lying on her back for the whole process.

Additional maternity leave (AML) This starts on the day after the Ordinary Maternity Leave (OML) period finishes, which is 26 weeks from the date you first went on leave. You can take up to 26 weeks of additional maternity leave.

Amniotic fluid The fluid within the amniotic sac which surrounds your baby. It is made up of mainly water with electrolytes, proteins, carbohydrates, fats, and urea, all of which aid in the growth of the foetus.

Amniotic sac The special membrane that surrounds the baby while it develops and is filled with amniotic fluid. Once the membrane breaks, it means your waters have broken and you've gone into labour.

Anaemia When the body lacks a sufficient amount of iron, which is needed for red blood cells. It can cause iron-deficiency anaemia, leading to tiredness and shortness of breath.

Analgesic An analgesic is a type of drug that provides pain relief. They include paracetamol and non-steroidal anti-inflammatory drugs such as ibuprofen.

Anomaly scan A scan given to a pregnant woman at 20 weeks (or sometimes between 18 and 22 weeks) to check her baby's development and the position of the placenta.

Apgar score Each newborn is checked one minute and five minutes after birth and given a score out of 10 known as an Apgar score. The midwife is checking skin colour, reflexes, heart rate, muscle tone and breathing.

Baby blues Feeling low and weepy in the days immediately after birth. It's usually caused by fluctuations in hormones and doesn't normally last longer than a week.

Beta human chorionic gonadotropin (HCG) A hormone released during pregnancy – it's what is detected when you take a pregnancy test.

Braxton hicks A tightening of the uterus muscles during pregnancy. They are a type of practise contraction, but not a sign of true labour.

Breech position When your baby is positioned with his head at the top of your uterus and his bottom at the opening to it.

Bromelain A protein found in pineapple which is thought to help soften the cervix in preparation for labour.

Cervix The opening to the uterus, which will dilate to allow your baby through when you give birth.

Colostrum A milky substance that provides all the nutrients and fluid that your newborn needs in the early days after birth, as well as lots of antibodies to protect your baby.

Diabetes A condition where your blood sugar levels become too high. In pregnancy, it is known as gestational diabetes, but will often disappear after your baby is born.

Down's Syndrome A genetic condition that is caused by the presence of an extra copy of chromosome 21, which can cause physical and mental disabilities.

Deep vein thrombosis (DVT) When a blood clot gets stuck in a vein in your body. The risk increases during pregnancy because your blood is more likely to clot to prevent blood loss during birth.

Edwards' Syndrome A genetic condition caused by the presence of an extra copy of chromosome 18, which can cause major brain abnormalities. Babies who have the syndrome are unlikely to survive longer than a few days.

Embryo When a fertilized egg starts to develop it changes from a zygote – a collection of cells – into an embryo. In humans, an embryo is considered to be between the first and eighth week of pregnancy.

Endometrium The lining of the womb which is shed each month during a period. During pregnancy, the fertilized egg implants itself into the endometrium and develops into a baby.

Endorphins Chemicals released during exercise and also during labour which have a naturally analgesic effect on pain in the body.

Entonox Entonox is a colourless, odourless gas made up of half oxygen and half nitrous oxide. It's also known as 'gas and air', or laughing gas.

Epidermis The top layer of skin cells.

Epidural A regional anaesthetic injected into your back to numb pain during labour via a thin tube called a catheter.

Episiotomy A cut made on the perineum – the tissue between the vagina and anus – during birth to help the baby be born more easily.

External cephalic version When a doctor attempts to turn a breech baby so that it is facing head down by manipulating your bump. It can be done from 36 weeks pregnant onwards.

Fallopian tube A tube that connects your ovary to your uterus. Each month an egg will travel down the fallopian tube. If it is fertilized, it will embed into the uterus and develop into a baby.

Foetal alcohol syndrome (FAS) Drinking too much alcohol during pregnancy can lead to FAS, which is characterized by specific mental and physical disabilities.

Foetus The medical term used to describe your growing baby from the second month of pregnancy until birth.

Folic acid An important B vitamin needed during pregnancy for the proper development of your baby, and the prevention of spina bifida. You should take 400mg per day while trying for a baby and for at least the first 12 weeks of pregnancy.

Follicle stimulating hormone (FSH) This is a hormone released by the pituitary gland which stimulates the release of an egg from the ovary each month.

Gestational diabetes Gestational diabetes happens when you have too much sugar in your blood during pregnancy. It's caused because hormones make the insulin in your body (which is responsible for controlling blood sugar levels) less responsive.

Group B streptococcus A type of bacteria which lives in the gut and vagina. It can occasionally be passed onto your baby during birth, and on rare occasions causes a serious infection. GBS infections can be prevented through antibiotics if it's picked up before labour begins.

Haem and non-haem iron There are two types of iron – haem and non-haem. Haem iron is found in meat and non-haem is found in foods of vegetable origin.

Haemoglobin The molecule in red blood cells that carries oxygen from the lungs. It is made from iron, and low haemoglobin levels (caused by a lack of iron) can cause anaemia.

Hibitane An obstetric cream used during internal examinations.

Hypnotherapy A method of relaxation, breathing and a way of focusing the mind. Hypnotherapy techniques form the key part of hypnobirthing.

Hyperemesis gravidarum Extreme sickness that occurs at any point during the day or night and for most of your pregnancy. It can cause severe dehydration, weight loss and hospitalisation.

Hypnobirthing A method of hypnotherapy used during pregnancy which entails using specific language alongside relaxation techniques to put you back in control of labour and reduce fear and pain.

Induction If a baby goes overdue (usually by at least a week), the mother will receive an induction, where drugs are given to stimulate contractions and start labour.

Iodine A mineral found in shellfish and plant foods which is needed to help in the development of your baby's brain and nervous system.

L-arginine An amino-acid that helps to boost male and female fertility by increasing blood flow to the reproductive organs and support sperm production.

Lanugo The fine, downy hair that covers your baby's body while in the womb. It helps to hold vernix in place and usually drops out before birth, or immediately afterwards.

Listeria A bacteria that is sometimes found in un-pasteurised dairy products, soft or mould-ripened cheeses, pâté and uncooked or under-cooked meat. It can cause listeriosis – a type of food poisoning that can be dangerous for your baby.

Luteinising hormone A hormone that is released, along with follicle stimulating hormone (FSH), by the pituitary gland. It stimulates the egg follicle to make and release oestrogen into the body.

Meconium Your baby's first bowel movement. It's made up of the contents of your baby's intestines and is a sticky, dark green substance.

Menstrual cycle A month-long process controlled by hormones that forms part of your reproductive system. If sexual intercourse doesn't happen at the right time, you will menstruate and the cycle will begin again.

Obstetrician A doctor that specializes in pregnancy and birth.

Obstetric cholestasis A pregnancy condition that affects your liver. It causes itching – specifically on the palms of your hands and soles of your feet.

Oestrogen A female hormone produced by the ovaries, which is responsible for regulating your reproductive cycle, and released by the placenta in pregnant women to maintain their pregnancy.

Ovulation When an egg is released from an ovary and begins to travel down the fallopian tube.

Oxytocin A hormone produced by the hypothalamus – an area in the brain – that stimulates the womb to start contracting and for labour to begin. It also helps to stimulate milk production for breastfeeding, and is released during sex and when we hug, which is why it's often called 'the cuddle hormone'.

Parasympathetic nervous system This system is responsible for controlling the bodily processes that are not under our own voluntary control, for example digesting food after we've eaten, or breathing.

Paediatrician A doctor that specializes in the health of babies and young children.

Patau's Syndrome A genetic condition caused by the presence of an extra copy of chromosome 13, which can cause major brain abnormalities. Babies who have the syndrome are unlikely to survive longer than a few days.

Pelvic floor muscles A sling of muscles that holds internal organs such as your bladder and uterus in place, and also helps to control the flow of your urine. Having weak pelvic floor muscles can be linked to incontinence.

Pelvis The pelvis is a sturdy ring of bone that is found at the bottom of the torso. It brings together the tailbone end of the spine and anchors the two hipbones in place.

Perineal massage Massaging the perineum – the area of skin between the vagina and anus – is thought to help make it stretchy and less liable to tear during childbirth.

Pethidine A painkiller offered as an injection during labour. It is anti-spasmodic and can also help you to relax. It is usually administered by a midwife.

Pica An intense craving which can occur in pregnancy to eat inedible products such as coal, paper, chalk or soil.

Pituitary gland A tiny gland (about the size of a pea) found in the head next to the brain which is responsible for releasing hormones including many responsible for reproduction.

Placenta An organ attached to the lining of the womb which delivers nutrients to your baby via the umbilical cord. It has its own blood supply which is separate to the mother's, but is also able to move nutrients and waste products between the mother and baby.

Placenta praevia When the placenta sits either partially or completely over the cervix – the opening to the uterus.

Polycystic ovary syndrome A condition that can affect a woman's ovaries, causing cysts to appear on them, and triggering a surge in male hormones (androgens) which can cause a range of side effects including irregular periods, excess hair growth and acne.

Pre-eclampsia A condition marked by high blood pressure and high levels of protein in your urine. If undiagnosed, it can lead to eclampsia, an extremely dangerous condition that can cause problems for mum and baby.

Prenatal depression Feelings of extreme sadness, anxiety and isolation which can occur during pregnancy.

Progesterone A female hormone produced by the corpus luteum, a part of the ovarian follicle that matures an egg each month. Once the egg is fertilized and the placenta starts to grow, it will take over the production of progesterone.

Prostaglandins Hormones created by a chemical process in the body. They help to stimulate the contraction of your uterus in labour. Manufactured forms of prostaglandins are given to kick-start labour if you go overdue.

Pudendal block The injection of an anaesthetic into the pudendal canal, which houses the pudendal nerve. It's done through your vagina just before birth to numb the area and make delivery less painful.

Relaxin A hormone released during pregnancy by the ovaries and placenta, which relaxes ligaments in the body so that the pelvis can widen to allow your baby out, as well as soften the cervix.

Rhesus status The status of your blood type – you can be either rhesus positive or rhesus negative. Your rhesus factor is determined by your genes.

Show A mucus-like discharge which appears just as your labour is starting. It is actually what plugs up the cervix during pregnancy to prevent bacteria entering the uterus, and falls away as your cervix starts to dilate.

Spina bifida A condition where the spine of a baby does not develop during pregnancy. A lack of folic acid in the first few months of pregnancy can increase your risk of spina bifida.

Surfactant Surfactant is a fatty substance that coats the inside or lining of the air sacs (alveoli) in the lungs of your growing baby and keeps them open, stopping them from collapsing. It's produced in the last few weeks of pregnancy.

Sweep When your midwife runs her fingers around your cervix to try and separate the membranes of your amniotic sac from it and trigger labour.

TENS machine A machine which releases pulses of electrical energy through pads attached to your back to help ease pain in labour by intercepting some of the pain signals trying to reach your brain. TENS stands for transcutaneous electrical nerve stimulation.

Thyroid disorder A thyroid disorder such as hyperthyroidism (over-active thyroid) can affect your fertility. The condition is caused where there is too much thyroid hormone in your body.

Transvaginal probe Used for ultrasounds, a transvaginal probe is a thin tube inserted into the vagina which can produce an ultrasound scan of your baby.

Ultrasound A type of scan produced when sound waves bounce off body tissues to produce an image of your baby. Ultrasound waves cannot pass through bone, air or gas.

Umbilical cord The tube that links your baby to your placenta and provides it with all the nutrients it needs, as well as removing the baby's waste products. The cord is cut after birth and eventually shrivels up, forming your baby's belly button.

Ventouse A machine that assists in the delivery of your baby. A suction cap on the ventouse is attached to your baby's head and a vacuum applied to help pull your baby out.

Vernix A waxy, white substance that you may see on your baby's skin after birth. It's made up of sebum (skin oil) and skin cells and is designed to protect the skin while in the womb.

Zinc A mineral found in meat, dairy and nuts. It plays an essential role in the construction of your baby's cells and DNA during pregnancy. It's also needed for healthy sperm production.

Zygote When a sperm fertilizes an egg, it becomes known as a zygote. Once the egg starts to divide and multiply it changes into a morula, a blastocyst and then finally an embryo.

MEET THE EXPERTS

Hannah Fox is a health journalist and writer with five years of experience in the pregnancy and parenting sector, including four years as a writer at *Mother&Baby* magazine. She has also written for numerous other health and wellbeing titles and websites including *Healthy*, *Women's Health UK* and *Unforgettable.org*.

Dr Petra Boynton specializes in research on sex and relationship health and runs the 'From Bump To Grind' project talking about sex and relationships for those trying to conceive, who are pregnant or who have children (www.facebook.com/groups/frombumptogrind).

Dr Ellie Cannon is a GP and author and is widely quoted in magazines, TV and radio on health matters, particularly those relating to pregnancy, parenting and diet (www.drellie.co.uk).

Shreelata Datta is a Consultant Obstetrician and Gynaecologist at King's College Hospital, London. She has written numerous articles, letters and books on Obstetrics and Gynaecology and is currently Joint Lead for Undergraduate Obstetrics and Gynaecology at King's College Medical School.

Dr Joanna Helcke is an expert in pregnancy and postnatal Pilates and winner of the 2014 FitPro Award for Excellence in Fitness. She is the creator of the first ever week-by-week online pregnancy fitness system (www.joannahelcke.com).

Fiona Kacz-Boulton is a fertility specialist, author, public speaker and leading fertility yoga teacher. She is the founder of Awakening Fertility, a specialist fertility programme that uses a range of professionals to help you live a more fertile lifestyle (www.awakeningfertility.com).

Helen Taylor qualified as a Registered Midwife in 1994 and worked for the NHS for 15 years, gaining valuable experience in all aspects of midwifery care. In 2009 she set up her independent midwifery company, Midwife Care (www.midwifecare.co.uk).

Mia Scotland is a clinical psychologist, hypnobirthing expert and birth doula (yourbirthright.co.uk), having trained with the reputable Michel Odent – a famous name in the birthing field. She has a passion for the psychology of birth, and understanding how good preparation is key to a good birth.

Charlotte Stirling-Reed is a registered nutrition consultant and founder of SR Nutrition (www.srnutrition.co.uk). Charlotte's main areas of interest include baby weaning, fussy eating and nutrition during pregnancy. She regularly provides expert comment for print and radio.

Mother&Baby is the UK's No. 1 Pregnancy, Baby and Toddler Magazine – and the home of all the latest expert advice covering every aspect of becoming a mum. *Mother&Baby* is sold in the UK, Eire, Australia, China, Croatia, Indonesia, Poland, Serbia, Singapore, Turkey, India and beyond. Find out more about *Mother&Baby* at www.motherandbaby.co.uk.

FURTHER RESOURCES

American Pregnancy Association
Health organization committed to promoting reproductive and pregnancy wellness through education, support, advocacy, and community awareness.
www.americanpregnancy.org

Antenatal Results and Choices
National charity helping parents and healthcare professionals through antenatal screening and its consequences.
www.arc-uk.org
Email: info@arc-uk.org
345 City Road, London, EC1V 1LR
Tel: 020 7713 7356

Association of Breastfeeding Mothers
Charity providing help, support and counselling to new mothers who wish to breastfeed.
www.abm.me.uk
Email: counselling@abm.me.uk
Tel: 0300 330 5453

Association for Postnatal Illness
Charity providing support to mothers suffering from postnatal illness by increasing public awareness of the illness and encouraging research into its cause and nature.
www.apni.org
Email: info@apni.org
145 Dawes Road,
Fulham,
London, SW6 7EB
Tel: 0207 386 0868

Australian Breastfeeding Association
Australia's largest breastfeeding information and support service.
www.breastfeeding.asn.au
1818–1822 Malvern Road, Malvern, East Vic, 3145
Tel: 1800 686 268

Awakening Fertility
Fertility programme run by Fiona Kacz-Boulton to aid couples trying to get pregnant.
www.awakeningfertility.com
The Harley Street Fertility Clinic, 134 Harley Street, W1G 7JY

Birth.co.au
Online resource for conception, pregnancy, labour, birth and newborn advice and community for women based in Australia.
www.birth.com.au

Birth Trauma Association
Charity which supports women suffering from Postnatal Post Traumatic Stress Disorder (PTSD) or birth trauma.
www.birthtraumaassociation.org.uk
PO Box 671, Ipswich, Suffolk IP1 9AT

Bliss
Charity supporting babies and their parents who are born premature.
www.bliss.org.uk
2nd Floor, Chapter House, 18–20 Crucifix Lane, London SE1 3JW
Tel: 0500 618140

Department for Work & Pensions
For information on maternity leave rights and benefits.
www.gov.uk/government/organisations/
department-for-work-pensions

Gingerbread
Charity providing support and information for single parents.
www.gingerbread.org.uk
520 Highgate Studios, 53–79 Highgate Road, London, NW5 1TL
Tel: 0808 802 0925

Home Start
Home-Start is a national family support charity that helps parents to build better lives for their children.
www.home-start.org.uk
The Home-Start Centre, 8–10 West Walk, Leicester, LE1 7NA

International Confederation of Midwives
International Confederation of Midwives aims to strengthen Midwives Associations and to advance the profession of midwifery globally by promoting autonomous midwives as the most appropriate caregivers for childbearing women.
www.internationalmidwives.org

Independent Midwife UK
Membership organisation and database for independent midwives in the UK.
www.imuk.org.uk
Email: info@imuk.org.uk
292 Ashley Down Road Bristol BS7 9BQ
Tel: 0300 111 0105

La Leche League GB
Providing information and support for breastfeeding mothers.
www.laleche.org.uk
Tel: 0845 120 2918

Midwife Care
Independent Midwifery service run by Helen Taylor
www.midwifecare.co.uk

Mother&Baby.co.uk
The website of *Mother&Baby* magazine and a source of useful information, product reviews and support.
www.motherandbaby.co.uk

National Childbirth Trust
Charity offering information and support in pregnancy, birth and early parenthood, including prenatal and postnatal courses.
www.nct.org.uk
0300 330 0700

Royal College of Obstetricians and Gynaecologists
Provides information, clinical guidelines, support and a network for professionals and women to receive the gynaecological and obstetric care they need.
www.rcog.org.uk
27 Sussex Place, Regent's Park, London, NW1 4RG, UK
Tel: 020 7772 6200

SR Nutrition
Consultancy run by Charlotte Stirling-Reed
providing advice and guidance on adult, child
and prenatal and postnatal nutrition.
www.srnutrition.co.uk
Email: info@srnutrition.co.uk
Tel: 0781 44 14 541

Tommy's
Charity that funds research into miscarriage,
premature birth and stillbirth.
www.tommys.org
Email: mailbox@tommys.org
Nicholas House, 3 Laurence Pountney Hill,
London, EC4R 0BB
Tel: 0207 398 3400

**Twins And Multiple Births Association
(TAMBA)**
Tamba is a UK based charity helping people who
are having or have had twins or multiple births.
www.tamba.org.uk
Email: enquiries@tamba.org.uk
Manor House, Church Hill, Aldershot, Hants,
GU12 4JU
Tel: 01252 332 344

Wellbeing of Women
Wellbeing of Women is the charity dedicated
to improving the health of women and babies
across the UK.
www.wellbeingofwomen.org.uk
Email: hello@wellbeingofwomen.org.uk
First Floor, Fairgate House, 78 New Oxford
Street, London, WC1A 1HB
Tel: 020 3697 7000

Working Families
A charity that helps working parents and carers
and their employers find a better balance
between responsibilities at home and work.
Their Legal Helpline gives parents and carers
advice on employment rights such as maternity
and paternity leave and parental leave.
www.workingfamilies.org.uk
Email: advice@workingfamilies.org.uk
Working Families, Cambridge House,
1 Addington Square, London, SE5 0HF
Tel: 0300 012 0312

Your Birth Right
Service run by clinical psychologist, doula and
hypnobirthing expert Mia Scotland offering
classes, advice and support in these areas.
www.yourbirthright.co.uk
Email: info@yourbirthright.co.uk
Tel: 0845 868 5904

Zest4LifeUK
Prenatal and postnatal fitness classes and
information run by fitness expert Joanna Helcke.
5 Burnaston Way, Loughborough, Leicestershire,
LE11 2HZ
www.joannahelcke.com
Email: hello@joannahelcke.com
Tel: 078999 38032

INDEX

An Hachette UK Company
www.hachette.co.uk

First published in Great Britain in 2016 by
Hamlyn, a division of
Octopus Publishing Group Ltd
Carmelite House
50 Victoria Embankment
London EC4Y 0DZ
www.octopusbooks.co.uk

ISBN 978 0 60063 215 3

A CIP catalogue record for this book is available
from the British Library.

Printed and bound in China

10 9 8 7 6 5 4 3 2 1

All reasonable care has been taken in the
preparation of this book but the information
it contains is not intended to take the place of
treatment by a qualified medical practitioner.

Before making any changes in your health
regime, always consult a doctor. While all the
therapies detailed in this book are completely
safe if done correctly, you must seek professional
advice if you are in any doubt about any medical
condition. Any application of the ideas and
information contained in this book is at the
reader's sole discretion and risk.

Publishing Director Stephanie Jackson
Editor Pauline Bache
Copy-editor Jemima Dunne
Designer Abigail Read and Jaz Bahra
Illustrator Abigail Read
Senior Production Manager Pete Hunt

Octopus Publishing Group would like to thank
Claire Irvin, Busola Evans, Hannah Fox, Dr Petra
Boynton, Dr Ellie Cannon, Shreelata Datta,
Dr Joanna Helcke, Fiona Kacz-Boulton, Helen
Taylor, Mia Scotland and Charlotte Stirling-Reed
for their contributions to this book.

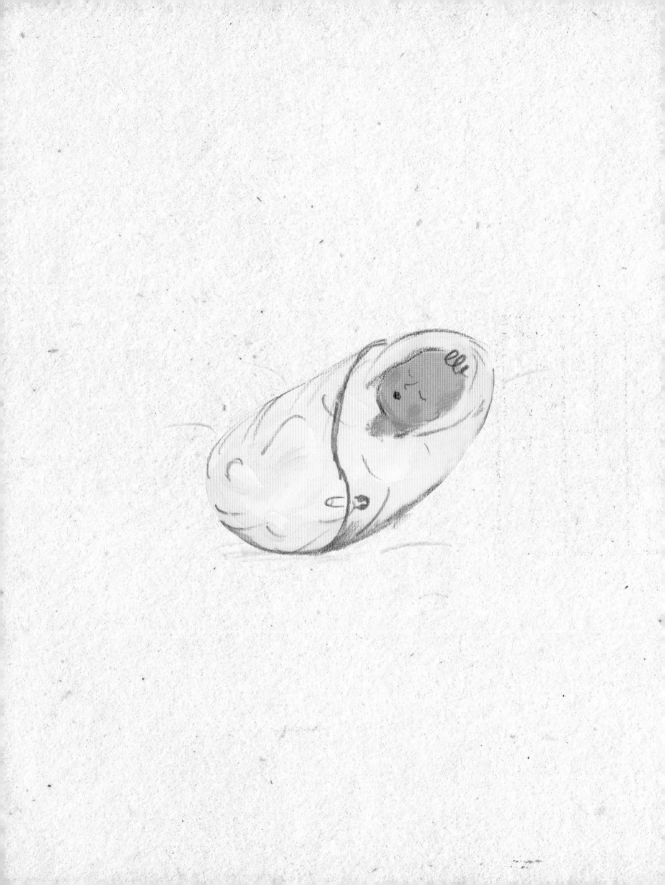